The Complete MRCGP
Study Guide

Sarah Gear

Foreword by

Professor Steve Field

Regional Postgraduate Dean, West Midlands Deanery
Chairman, Education Network
Royal College of General Practitioners

RADCLIFFE MEDICAL PRESS

Radcliffe Medical Press Ltd
18 Marcham Road
Abingdon
Oxon OX14 1AA
United Kingdom

www.radcliffe-oxford.com
The Radcliffe Medical Press electronic catalogue and online ordering facility.
Direct sales to anywhere in the world.

British Library Cataloguing in Publication Data

A catalogue record for this book is available from the British Library.

ISBN 1 85775 865 X

Typeset by Acorn Bookwork Ltd, Salisbury
Printed and bound by TJ International Ltd, Padstow, Cornwall

Contents

Foreword

The MRCGP examination is the 'Gold Standard' assessment of GP Registrars. It has been devised by the Royal College of General Practitioners as an assessment of the knowledge, skills and attitudes appropriate to the general practitioner on completion of vocational training. It is pitched at a higher level than that of Summative Assessment, but it is a level that should be attainable by all GP Registrars.

The MRCGP Examination continues to evolve and develop while retaining its reputation as one of the most valid and reliable examinations in British medicine. The introduction of the 'Single Route' for the assessment of communication skills has, however, proved very popular with GP Registrars undergoing Summative Assessment at the end of their training. A majority now submit video tapes through the 'Single Route', an increasing number are taking all of the Examination's modules with a tremendous pass rate of over 80%. The RCGP membership is rising and there are many people calling for the MRCGP Examination to become the end point assessment for all GP Registrars.

While more and more GP Registrars are taking the MRCGP Examination, there are also increasing numbers of established GPs choosing to take the Examination in order to become a Trainer or purely as a quality marker. Many choose the examination route over the Membership by Assessment route.

The Complete MRCGP Study Guide will help both groups of doctors in their pursuit of the 'Gold Standard'. It is the most up-to-date MRCGP revision book on the market. It is written by a young GP who has recently excelled as a candidate herself. She has learned many lessons from her experiences that will help the reader; it is packed full of useful information, ideas and advice that I am sure will help increase the pass rate even more!

Sarah has kept me informed of progress during the book's evolution and I have been really impressed by how she set about the task and am delighted with the outcome. I commend it to you, the reader, and look forward to you joining me as a member of the College.

Professor Steve Field
Regional Postgraduate Dean, West Midlands Deanery
Chairman, Education Network
Royal College of General Practitioners
November 2003

About the author

Dr Sarah L Gear graduated in 1995 from Manchester Medical School. She undertook SHO posts followed by the GP vocational training scheme at the North Staffordshire Royal Infirmary in Stoke-on-Trent, qualifying as a GP in August 2001 and successfully gaining the MRCGP the same year.

In April 2002, she became a principal at her former training practice in Madeley near Crewe. Although working half-time in practice she also does sessional family planning and some locum work.

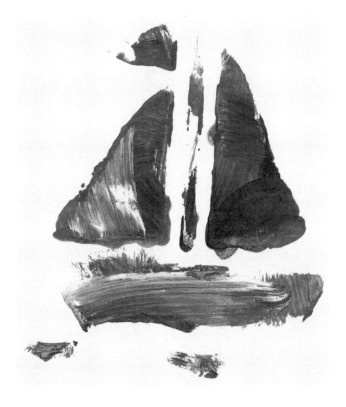

Nick Gear, aged 1.

Introduction

- You don't need to know everything (you cannot possibly).

- It is easier if what you are learning is topical/relevant.

- It is not how much you know, but how you apply that knowledge, that matters.

- Hot topics form only a small part of the exam, whether it is the MRCGP or summative assessment.

- You generally do not need to quote specific references.

Thus we have established that the exam is not about knowing everything. Let's face it, there would be little point in knowing all about the treatment of Indian visceral leishmaniasis for day-to-day general practice. Many studies that influence general practice today were completed years ago. Being able to regurgitate a textbook, hot topics or anything else, does not mean that you have got the exam cracked. And it certainly does not make you a better doctor.

The College Website (www.rcgp.org.uk) is a must. Even if you have sat the exam before, you must read the rules again – they can change, so don't be caught out.

Part of the groundwork is to speak to as many people as possible about their learning techniques and approach for the MRCGP. You will find that in the majority of cases people will identify a topic ('learning need') and read around it from, say, a textbook. Then they might do a Medline search for current review articles or look in *Clinical Evidence* to check whether there is any new revolutionary information that might change the way they would tackle the given subject (i.e. the way they practise).

The more enlightened doctors manage to keep up to date with the journals and comics, do their own video analysis and even have a mentor. This would form part of a personal development plan (PDP). By thinking about what you would want to achieve in general practice from early on in your career, you will be able to maximise the benefit that you gain from your hospital jobs.

To be a medically competent GP you need to be well read (a true generalist) and have an open, sensible approach to acquiring knowledge that will fill in any gaps. You need to be able to work as part of a team (you will be part of the primary healthcare team, not to mention the doctor–patient partnership), and you need to be open to ethical and cultural ideas and beliefs. That's all just for starters!

In this book I have covered the main medical topics that are fundamental to general practice. This is not meant to provide a comprehensive coverage of aetiology, pathophysiology, investigations and treatments – quite the opposite. I assume that if you are not up to speed and need to recap, you will be able to access this information easily. I have incorporated current treatment issues, National Service Frameworks, the latest research, questions, etc. It is all clearly referenced and the issues are not clouded by my personal opinions, as the whole point of postgraduate learning is to formulate your own. Having said that, where it seemed important to do so, I have included the opinions of published authors from the journals.

All of this is to save you the colossal amount of time that you would otherwise need to prepare for the exam.

Sarah Gear
November 2003
gear@doctors.org.uk

How to use this book

Probably the worst thing you could do at this stage is to try and plough through from beginning to end – you would never make it (this is not a challenge), and even if you did, you would be unlikely to remember much of it.

Use the book as a starting point, a guide or for summing up to ensure that you are as well read as you think you are. Flick through and get a handle on the layout and what is included. No doubt there will be parts you know inside out, so do not be tempted to spend too much time here, but move on. Scribble comments and questions, highlight text, use Post-it notes, or completely deface it if necessary. Do whatever you like, but make sure that it works for you.

As you go through the different sections, think not only of possible questions that the examiners might set, but also if you had to teach the subject how you would explain the various issues. Write down the questions you come up with and use them for revision (e.g. in a study group).

With regard to the exam-style questions, each part explains what is involved and suggests ways of tackling them (e.g. against the clock, in pairs, etc.). All of the answers are comprehensive but not exhaustive. As you get used to the techniques and increase your knowledge base, there will be points that you feel are important which I have not included. Keep them as part of your answer.

No book will ever cover everything you need to know, but this one encompasses a huge amount. I hope you find it an indispensable guide to both your GP registrar year and the MRCGP.

General practice is a fantastic career. The MRCGP is not yet essential (unless you want to become a trainer), but it is a worthwhile exam to work for. You will gain an incredible amount from it if you are willing to put in the time and effort. Enjoy, and good luck!

Mum, Dad and My Guys

You can never repay the sun
for its gift of light

Part I

Coronary heart disease (CHD)

National Service Framework for CHD

Launched in March 2000 (doh.gov.uk/nsf/coronary.htm), this is a follow-on from the White Paper *Saving Lives: Our Healthier Nation*, in which CHD was set out as a priority.

It is a 10-year plan which:

- aims to reduce death from CHD and stroke by 40% by the year 2010 in people up to 75 years of age
- emphasises the need to provide structured systematic care.

Since its launch, statin prescribing has doubled.

There are 12 standards, but the following priorities are highlighted:

- smoking cessation advice
- CHD register in primary care
- rapid assessment chest pain clinic
- faster treatment for myocardial infarction, and improved secondary prevention
- more heart operations/revascularisation.

Standards that mainly affect primary care

- Standard 2 – smoking cessation advice
- Standards 3 and 4 – these cover secondary prevention followed by primary prevention:
  - comprehensive CHD register for audit purposes
  - development of protocols and guidelines (these need to be agreed at practice level, primary care group/trust level and across primary, secondary and tertiary care)
- Standard 11 – heart failure and palliative care for people with CHD – we are responsible for arranging appropriate investigations to confirm diagnosis and then offering appropriate treatment.

Workload issues

These include the following:

- identifying patients and maintaining registers
- regular audit (every 3 months)

- practice time (meetings, clinics, following protocols and guidelines, etc.)

- treating the patient/pharmacology.

○ (2001) GP workload implications of the NSF for CHD: cross-sectional survey. *BMJ.* **323**: 269–70 (*see also* the accompanying editorial).
This study found a significant workload. It was estimated that for 1000 men aged 40–55 years in a practice, that practice would need four full-time nurses for 18 months to record data and tackle the necessary issues. Given adequate resources, risk factors for hypertension, lipids and diabetic/HbA_{1C} risk could be reduced.

If we as GPs are to be held accountable (which we will be), then we need adequate staffing with appropriate training.

Interestingly, *Health Statistics Quarterly* (www.nationalstatistics.gov.uk) gives weight to the argument that GPs do not need Government guidance to keep their practice up to date. Prescribing habits had changed appropriately prior to the publication of the National Service Framework (compare with ACE inhibitors in congestive cardiac failure).

National Service Framework for Coronary Heart Disease – Standards

Reducing heart disease in the population
1 The NHS and partner agencies should develop, implement and monitor policies that reduce the prevalence of coronary risk factors in the population, and reduce the inequalities in risks of developing heart disease.
2 The NHS and partner agencies should contribute to a reduction in the prevalence of smoking in the local population.

Preventing CHD in high-risk patients in primary care
3 General practitioners and primary care teams should identify all people with established cardiovascular disease and offer them comprehensive advice and appropriate treatment to reduce their risks.
4 General practitioners and primary care teams should identify all people at significant risk of cardiovascular disease who have not yet developed symptoms, and offer them appropriate advice and treatment to reduce their risks.

Heart attacks: acute myocardial infarction and other acute coronary syndromes
5 People with symptoms of a possible heart attack should receive help from an individual equipped with and appropriately trained in the use of a defibrillator within 8 minutes of calling for help, to maximise the benefits of resuscitation should it be necessary.
6 People thought to be suffering from a heart attack should be assessed professionally and, if indicated, receive aspirin. Thrombolysis should be given within 60 minutes of calling for professional help.
7 NHS trusts should put in place agreed protocols/systems of care so that people admitted to hospital with proven heart attacks are appropriately assessed and offered treatments of proven clinical and cost-effectiveness to reduce their risk of disability and death.

Stable angina

8 People with symptoms of angina or suspected angina should receive appropriate investigation and treatment to relieve their pain and reduce their risk of coronary events.

Revascularisation

9 People with angina that is increasing in frequency or severity should be referred to a cardiologist urgently, or for those at greatest risk, as an emergency.

10 NHS trusts should put in place hospital-wide systems of care so that patients with suspected or confirmed CHD receive timely and appropriate investigation and treatment to relieve their symptoms and reduce their risk of subsequent coronary events.

Heart failure and palliative care for people with CHD

11 Doctors should arrange for people with suspected heart failure to be offered appropriate investigations (e.g. electrocardiography, echocardiography) that will confirm or refute the diagnosis and, where this is confirmed, offer the treatment most likely to both relieve their symptoms and reduce the risk of death.

Cardiac rehabilitation and secondary prevention of CHD

12 NHS trusts should put in place agreed protocols/systems of care so that prior to leaving hospital, people admitted suffering from CHD have been invited to participate in a multidisciplinary programme of secondary prevention and cardiac rehabilitation. The aim of the programme will be to reduce their risk of subsequent cardiac problems and to promote their return to a full and normal life.

Hypertension

This is bread-and-butter general practice.

○ British Hypertension Society Guidelines. (1999) *J Hum Hypertens.* **13**: 569–92 and *BMJ.* **319**: 630–5.

It is important to know these guidelines, which are based on the HDT trial.

○ (1998) Effects of intensive BP lowering and low-dose aspirin in patients with hypertension: principal results of the Hypertension Optimal Treatment (HOT) randomised trial. *Lancet.* **351**: 1755–62.
This trial included 18790 patients in 26 countries (with follow-up at 3.8 years on average), and it looked at outcomes in terms of major cardiovascular events. *Felodipine* (calcium-channel antagonist) was the baseline therapy.
   The lowest incidence of major cardiovascular events, a 30% reduction, occurred at a mean achieved diastolic blood pressure of 83 mmHg. For diabetes, the lowest incidence was found at a blood pressure of <80 mmHg.
   Daily addition of aspirin 75 mg reduced the risk of myocardial infarction by 36% in men, in well-controlled hypertension.

Summary of BHS Guidelines

- Give non-pharmacological advice to all hypertensives (and borderline hypertensives).

- Start antihypertensives in patients with:
  - *sustained systolic BP ≥ 160 mmHg*
  - *sustained diastolic BP ≥ 100 mmHg.*

- Treat borderline BP (140–159 mmHg/90–99 mmHg) if there is target organ damage, cardiovascular disease, diabetes or a 10-year risk >15%.

- Optimal BP targets are as follows:
  - systolic BP <140 mmHg
  - diastolic BP <85 mmHg.

  The minimum acceptable control for audit purposes is 150/90 mmHg, *and for diabetics it is 130/80 mmHg.*

- If there are no contraindications, first-line treatment is with thiazides or beta-blockers.

- Consider other drugs that reduce cardiovascular risk (e.g. aspirin if 10-year risk is >15%, and statins if 10-year risk is >30%).

○ (2001) Cardiovascular protection and blood pressure reduction. *Lancet.* **358**: 1305–6.
This meta-analysis of nine drug trials (involving 62 605 patients) showed little difference in the outcome of antihypertensive effects of diuretics, beta-blockers, calcium-channel blockers and ACE inhibitors. The emphasis was on the fact that it is the ultimate blood pressure control that is important.

○ (2002) Major outcomes in high-risk hypertensive patients randomised to ACEI or Ca-channel blockers vs. diuretics: the antihypertensive and lipid-lowering treatment to prevent heart attack trial (ALLHAT Trial). *JAMA.* **288**: 2981–97.
This multicentre randomised controlled trial involving 42 418 patients aged over 55 years confirmed the above meta-analysis. It was concluded that the most important factor in reducing risk and mortality is a reduction in blood pressure, not the actual drug used.

○ (2002) Cardiovascular morbidity and mortality in the losartan intervention for end-point reduction in hypertension study (LIFE): a randomised trial against atenolol. *Lancet.* **359**: 995–1003.
This study involved 9193 patients (aged 55–80 years) with essential hypertension (160–200/95–115 mmHg) and left ventricular hypertrophy (shown on ECG). There was a lower rate of new-onset diabetes with losartan (a difference of 25%), but no difference in the incidence of myocardial infarction between patients on losartan and those on atenolol (4%).
It was found that 4 years of treatment with either losartan or atenolol (randomised) was equally effective in lowering blood pressure. Losartan reduced the rates of fatal and non-fatal stroke (by 5% in patients on losartan and 7% in those on atenolol).

Blood-pressure-measuring devices

Most sphygmomanometers in general practice are not serviced and calibrated, which means that GPs may misclassify patients. The need for recalibration has been emphasised by the British Hypertension Society since 1986.

○ (2000) *Br J Gen Pract.* **50**: 725.
   This study found that several automated readings were more accurate than a single sphygmoman-ometer reading.

○ (2001) BP measuring devices: recommendations of the European Society of Hypertension. *BMJ.* **322**: 531–6.
   This is a rather dry read, emphasising recalibration in accordance with British Hypertension Society protocols and standards set by the US Association for the Advancement of Medical Instrumentation (AAMI).

Hypertension in the elderly

Half of all people aged over 60 years have hypertension. Several studies have provided evidence about treatment of hypertension in the elderly.

● *EWPHE (European Working Party on Hypertension in the Elderly).* In a study of 840 patients aged ⩾60 years and with BP > 160/90 mmHg, thiazide vs. placebo produced a significant reduction in cardiovascular mortality and death from myocardial infarction.

● *SHEP study (Systolic Hypertension in the Elderly Project).* In a study of 4736 patients aged ⩾60 years and with BP > 160/90 mmHg, thiazide vs. placebo (could switch to atenolol or reserpine if this was ineffective) caused a reduction in all major cardiovascular events (especially marked in the diabetic subgroup).

● *MRC and STOP H trials* have both confirmed the above findings.

British Hypertension Society guidelines recommend that drug treatment is of proven benefit up to 80 years of age, and that once started it should be continued. If hypertension is diagnosed after the age of 80 years, base the decision to treat on the clinical picture; thiazides are the preferred first-line therapy.

○ (2000) *Lancet.* **355**: 865.
   This meta-analysis looking at isolated systolic hypertension showed a correlation of mortality with wide pulse pressures (high systolic and low diastolic) as an indicator of atherosclerosis.

Heart failure

Represents a complex clinical syndrome characterised by abnormalities in LV function, neurohormonal regulation, exercise intolerance, shortness of breath, fluid retention and reduced longevity.

(Wilson, 1997)

Heart failure is not a diagnosis – you need to consider ischaemic heart disease, hypertension, cardiomyopathy, valvular heart disease, etc. There is a poor correlation between symptoms and signs when compared with echocardiographic findings. This is well recognised, and was discussed in the following articles.

o   (2000) *BMJ*. **320**: 220.

o   (2000) *Br J Gen Pract*. **50**: 50.

Heart failure has been targeted by *Standard 11* of the National Service Framework, as it is known that we under-diagnose and under-treat heart failure. It highlights the need for correct diagnosis and appropriate investigation.

- Prevalence is 3–20 per 1000 among the general population.

- Prevalence is 100 per 1000 in those over 65 years of age.

- Afro-Caribbeans over 65 years of age are at 2.5 times greater risk.

Diagnosis

The European Society of Cardiology's guidelines for diagnosis of heart failure are as follows.

- *Essential*: symptoms – shortness of breath, swollen ankles, fatigue *and* objective evidence of cardiac dysfunction at rest.

- *Non-essential*: response to treatment directed towards heart failure.

Diagnostic accuracy

- FINLAND Report: 32% of patients diagnosed with heart failure in primary care had definitive heart failure

- ECHOES study (Echocardiographic Heart of England Screening): 22% of patients with a diagnosis of heart failure had definitive impairment of left ventricular function.

o   (1994) Clinical diagnosis by hospital physicians is just as poor. *Br Heart J*. **72**: 584–7.
    If we were to refer everyone for echocardiography the system would be overwhelmed. It has been suggested that we refer patients whose ECG or chest X-ray is abnormal. Interestingly, the NSF stated that open-access echocardiography should have been available to all GPs by April 2002.

o   (2003) Barriers to accurate diagnosis and effective management of heart failure in primary care: qualitative study. *BMJ*. **326**: 196–200.
    This study identified three reasons why GPs had difficulty in diagnosing and managing heart failure:
    1   uncertainty about clinical practice
       –   diagnostic process – third heart sound, raised jugular venous pressure (especially in obese patients)
       –   availability and use of echocardiography services

– treatment issues
2 lack of awareness of relevant research evidence
3 influence of individual preferences and local organisational factors.

New York Heart Association (NYHA) grading of dyspnoea or angina

Grade	Criteria
1	Symptoms only occur on severe exertion; almost normal lifestyle possible
2	Symptoms occur on moderate exertion; patients have to avoid certain situations (e.g. carrying shopping up stairs)
3	Symptoms occur on mild exertion; activity is markedly restricted
4	Symptoms occur frequently, even at rest

Natriuretic peptides

Brain natriuretic peptide is found at high levels in patients with impaired left ventricular systolic function. As yet there are conflicting data from studies related to practical use, as there is a low positive predictive value. A role may develop for their use in helping to determine who to send for echocardiography.

The cost is around £25 per test.

Treatment of heart failure

In April 2000, the *Drug and Therapeutics Bulletin* reviewed treatment.

Diuretics

These are essential for symptomatic management (first-line treatment). Their long-term effect on mortality is not known, and it would be unethical to conduct a randomised controlled trial, given the known benefits of treatment.

- Potassium-sparing diuretics (e.g. amiloride).

- Spironolactone (competitive aldosterone inhibitor).

○ (1999) *NEJM*. **341**: 709–17.

○ (1999) *Lancet*. **341**: 709.
In the RALES trial (Randomised Aldactone Evaluation Study), 1663 patients with NYHA grade 4 disease who were already on an angiotensin converting enzyme (ACE) inhibitor and loop diuretic (i.e. severe heart failure) were randomised to receive spironolactone 25 mg/day or placebo. Improved mortality was observed, and hyperkalaemia was uncommon if a low dose (25 mg/day) was used.

ACE inhibitors

Trials have consistently shown prolonged survival, reversal of left ventricular hypertrophy and a reduced need for hospital admission due to left ventricular dysfunction.

Numbers needed to treat (NNT) quoted in different papers are as follows:

- for 1 year to prevent one death – 74 if ACE inhibitors alone are used
- for 1 year to prevent one death – 29 if ACE inhibitors plus beta-blocker are used.

An International Survey of the Management of Heart Failure in Primary Care was presented in September 2001. A total of 1000 GPs were questioned, and it was found that 90% were aware of the benefits of ACE inhibitors, 90% were sending patients for ECGs and 80% were sending patients for chest X-rays. About a third referred patients for echocardiography (services were thought to be inadequate). Although ACE inhibitors were being used, they were being given at inadequate doses. Only 19% of GPs were starting treatment with beta-blockers, and only 30% of patients under 70 years of age with heart failure were receiving them.

Thus as GPs our knowledge of heart failure is quite good, and we are starting to have success with ACE inhibitors, but we need to promote beta-blockers in a similar way.

- CONSENSUS I 1987 (Co-operative North Scandinavian Enalapril Study): this showed decreased mortality (with 20 mg enalapril bd) (with a follow-up period of 1 year) in patients with severe heart failure (NYHA grade 4).
- SOLVD (Study of Left Ventricular Dysfunction).

  ○ (1991) *NEJM*. **325**: 293–302.

  ○ (1992) *NEJM*. **327**: 685–91.
    This study showed benefits with enalapril 10 mg bd (with a follow-up period of 4 years). SOLVD-P confirmed that progression was slowed even if the patient was asymptomatic.

The following trials support the use of ACE inhibitors after myocardial infarction. There was a decrease in both mortality and progression of heart failure.

- SAVE (Survival and Ventricular Enlargement Trial)
  ○ (1992) *NEJM*.
- AIRE (Acute Infarction Ramipril Efficacy Study)
  ○ (1993) *Lancet*.
- TRACE (Trandalopril Cardiac Evaluation Study)
  ○ (1995) *NEJM*.

The results of the HOPE study (Heart Outcomes Prevention Evaluation study) suggest that everyone without contraindications should be on an ACE inhibitor.

  ○ (2000) *Lancet*. **355**: 253–9.

Beta-blockers

There is no longer an absolute contraindication. Beta-blockers are thought to work by their effects on the renin-angiotensin system and anti-arrhythmic properties. Over 20 randomised controlled trials have been conducted on 20 000 patients. The number needed to treat is 29 if beta-blockers and ACE inhibitors are used (to prevent one death over 1 year).

Beta-blockers are only indicated in moderate heart failure secondary to ischaemia (confirmed by echocardiography).

- CIBIS (Cardiac Insufficiency Bisoprolol Study): the results were not significant, but the trend was towards an improvement in survival.

- CIBIS II: this was superior to placebo with regard to mortality and morbidity (32%). The trial was stopped early because the results were so dramatic.

   ○ (2001) *Am Heart J*. **142**: 987–9.

- Carvedilol (USA): this was superior to placebo with regard to mortality and morbidity. The trial was stopped early.

   ○ (1996) *NEJM*. **334**: 1349–55 and (2003) *Lancet*. **362**: 7–13 (superior to metoprolol).

- MERIT-HF: metoprolol was superior to placebo for morbidity and mortality. The trial was stopped early.

   ○ (1999) *Lancet*. **353**: 2001–7.

Angiotensin II receptor antagonists

The following small randomised controlled trials have been conducted.

- ELITE (Evaluation of Losartan in the Elderly): this tolerability study of losartan vs. captopril in patients over 65 years of age suggested there was a benefit to patients who could not tolerate ACE inhibitors.

   ○ (1997) *Lancet*. **349**: 747–52.

- ELITE II: proved not to be superior to captopril with regard to survival. There was a confirmed better tolerability in this trial of 3152 patients.

   ○ (1999) *J Card Failure*. **5**: 146–54.

- Val-HeFT: in this trial of 366 patients who were not on ACE inhibitors, valsartan was used in addition, and there was a significant reduction in mortality.

   ○ (2002) *J Am Coll Cardiol*. **40**: 1414–21.

Digoxin

- RADIANCE (Randomised Assessment of Digoxin on Inhibitors of ACE).

- PROVED study (Prospective Randomised Study of Ventricular Failure and the Efficacy of Digoxin): both of these studies showed that digoxin prevented clinical worsening and improved symptoms.

- DIG (Digoxin Investigators Group): in this trial of 6800 patients who had heart failure but no atrial fibrillation, there was no decrease in mortality, but there was a symptomatic improvement.

Vasodilators

- V-HeFT I and II: in these trials of hydralazine and isosorbide dinitrate vs. placebo (I) or enalapril (II), there was improved mortality, but it was not as good as with enalapril (i.e. the alternative in patients with renal failure).

Multidisciplinary approaches to nutrition, patient counselling and education

There have been six small randomised controlled trials of highly selected patients. These showed reduced hospital admission rates, better education and improved quality of life.

- ○ (2001) *BMJ.* **323**: 715–18.
  This randomised controlled trial of specialist nurse intervention in heart failure showed that home-based intervention by nurses can reduce admissions. This is thought to be due to education, treatment and regular contact.

Lipids, statins and cardiovascular disease

Around 55% of the UK population have a total cholesterol concentration of >5.5 mmol/L, in 25% it is >6.5 mmol/L and in 5% it is >7.8 mmol/L.

Serum cholesterol levels can vary by up to 20% through the course of the day (i.e. any sample needs to be obtained while the patient is fasting).

Primary prevention evidence

- *AF/TexCAPS* (Air Force/Texas Coronary Atherosclerosis Prevention Study): primary prevention by placebo vs. lotorvostatin 20–40 mg was studied in 5608 middle-aged men and 997 women (with a (7-year follow-up). There was a 34% decrease in new events, which started to become evident after 6 months.

- *WOSCOPS* (West of Scotland Coronary Prevention Study): primary prevention was studied in high-risk male patients. There was a 22% decrease in mortality and a 25% decrease in coronary events.

- *ASCOT* (Anglo-Scandinavian Cardiac Outcomes Trial): this trial looked at the effect of adding atorvastatin to antihypertensive treatment in patients with a normal cholesterol concentration. It found a 30% reduction in myocardial infarction and stroke. The trial was stopped 2 years early and has yet to be published. There could be huge financial implications for the NHS.

Treatment in primary prevention is difficult despite the availability of risk assessment tools, especially when you consider potential cost. Diet and secondary causes should be looked at in the first instance. Treatment is advised (DTB, *BMJ*, NSF, etc.)

if the 10-year risk is >30%. If the 10-year risk is 15–30%, you need to take local advice with regard to resources, although patients would benefit. The number needed to treat (to prevent one death over 5 years) is 69.

Secondary prevention evidence

- *4S Study* (Scandinavian Simvastatin Survival Study): in this triple-blind Scandinavian study (94 centres) of 4444 patients aged 35–70 years (81.4% of whom were male) with coronary heart disease (angina or myocardial infarction), only 37% were on aspirin, and 57% were on beta-blockers. Simvastatin 20 mg vs. placebo (with a follow-up period of 5.4 years) decreased coronary events (42% reduction in mortality; relative risk, 0.58; CI, 0.46–0.73) and cardiovascular mortality (35%; relative risk, 0.65; CI, 0.52–0.8).

  ○ (1994) Randomised trial of cholesterol lowering in 4444 patients with CHD: the Scandinavian Simvastatin Survival Study. *Lancet*. **344**: 1383–9.

- *LIPID* (Long-Term Intervention with Pravastatin in IHD): in this study, 9000 patients with ischaemic heart disease were treated with placebo vs. pravastatin. There was a 25% decrease in mortality, cardiac events and procedures (6-year follow-up). A trial follow-up reinforced the initial findings.

  ○ (1995) *Am J Cardiol*. **76**: 474–9.

  ○ Trial follow-up: (2002) **352**: 1379-87.

- *CARE* (Cholesterol and Recurrent Events Trial): post-myocardial infarction patients were treated with pravastatin vs. placebo (5-year follow-up). There was a 22% decrease in mortality, 33% decrease in CHD and 20–31% decrease in stroke.

  ○ (1996) *NEJM*. **335**: 1001–9.

Statin treatment should be offered to all patients with atherosclerotic disease (with dietary advice, etc.) to reduce cholesterol levels to <5 mmol/L or by 30%, whichever is greater. The National Service Framework for CHD supports this.

The number needed to treat (to prevent one death over 5 years) is 16.

Statins underused by those who would benefit

Many people who would benefit from statins are not receiving them.

○ (2000) *BMJ*. **321**: 971–2.

○ (2001) Randomised trials of secondary prevention programmes in CHD: systematic review. *BMJ*. **323**: 957–62.
A total of 12 trials were conducted on 9803 patients with CHD. It was concluded that disease management programmes improve the process of care, reduce admissions and enhance quality of life. Disease management programmes include patient education, practice guidelines, appropriate consultations, supplies of drugs and ancillary services.

○ (2002) Heart Protection Study of cholesterol lowering with simvastatin in 20 536 high-risk individuals: a randomised placebo-controlled trial. *Lancet*. **360**: 7–20.

In this hospital-based UK study of people aged 40–80 years with cholesterol levels >3.5 mmol/L and an estimated 10-year risk of CHD of 40%, these patients had been diagnosed with coronary heart disease, other occlusive arterial disease, or diabetes (I and II), or had treated hypertension. It was found that simvastatin produced substantial benefits for a range of high-risk patients irrespective of the initial cholesterol concentration. It was also found that the drug was safe and well tolerated. Simvastatin 40 mg reduced myocardial infarction, cerebrovascular accidents and revascularisation by 25% (probably up to a third when corrected for compliance). In high-risk patients it would prevent 70–100 per 1000 cases. This could mean tripling the number of people on statins.

Role of plant stanols (e.g. Benecol and Flora Pro-Active)

○ (2000) *BMJ*. **320**: 861–4.
This meta-analysis of all randomised controlled trials showed that a 2 g daily intake of plant stanols resulted in a 9–14% reduction in LDL-cholesterol levels.

Primary prevention of cardiovascular disease

Risk assessment

Individuals are at increased risk of developing CVD if they are smokers, hypertensive, have dyslipidaemias or diabetes mellitus. Preventing CVD can be argued to be one of the most important tasks for GPs.

Absolute risk is the probability of developing CHD (non-fatal myocardial infarction or coronary death) over a defined period of time, and can be estimated using risk assessment charts. These help us to explain risks to the patient, which in turn empowers them to make informed choices. The information from the charts should not replace clinical judgement.

Most risk assessment tools are based on complex mathematics from the Framingham studies, although they are now relatively simple to use. They are designed for use in *primary prevention*. They are not for use in patients who have existing diseases which already put them at high risk, such as CHD, atherosclerotic disease, familial hypercholesterolaemia, inherited dyslipidaemia or renal dysfunction (including diabetic nephropathy).

The original Framingham study (named after a town in Massachusetts) was published in 1971 (*Ann Int Med*. **74**: 1–12), having looked for over 14 years at 2282 men and 2845 women, their lipid profiles and coronary heart disease risks. Since then a multitude of spin-off studies have been published relating to CHD.

○ (2000) Using the Framingham Model to predict heart disease in the UK: retrospective study. *BMJ*. **320**: 676–7.
This study has validated the data (i.e. it can be used to predict coronary risk in white men and women (but not ethnic minorities) in the UK).

Several prediction charts have been developed from this.

○ (2002) *Br J Gen Pract*. **52**: 135–7.
This study found that men with a positive family history had almost twice the risk of developing cardiovascular disease. The Framingham study does not account for familial risk.

Joint British Societies coronary risk prediction chart

This chart was produced by the British Cardiac, Hypertension, Hyperlipidaemia and Diabetic Associations. It distinguishes between diabetics and non-diabetics, men and women, and smokers and non-smokers. The graphs then depend upon systolic blood pressure, total cholesterol: HDL ratio and also a person's age.

It sounds complicated but it is simple to use (*see* the *British National Formulary* or *MIMS*).

New Zealand tables

These look at the 5-year risk and include the number needed to treat.

Sheffield tables

These look at the 10-year risk and break the estimates down into 15% and 30% risks.

SCORE

This is a project based on the meta-analysis of 12 studies in Europe (involving 250 000 people), as it is thought that the risk assessment tables based on Framingham overestimated the CHD risk. Individual risk charts will be tailor-made for a specific population.

Local variations on tables may be in operation (e.g. through biochemistry departments), and it is worth knowing about these.

Problems with tables

No system is perfect.

- Tables usually calculate a 10-year risk, and this becomes inaccurate with blood pressure and lifestyle changes over time, so you need to reassess periodically.

- They can be time-consuming to include opportunistically in a consultation (despite IT facilities).

- They do not always take into account ethnicity (which increases the risk by *c.* 1.5).

- They underestimate the risk if there is a strong family history of CHD below 65 years of age or hyperlipidaemia (in these cases you need to increase the risk estimate by a factor of 1.5).

Atrial fibrillation (AF)

AF is the commonest tachydysrhythmia diagnosed on ECG. It is important to diagnose, as it may be the first sign of heart disease and is an important risk factor for strokes. There is no known cause in 20–30% of cases.

The prevalence of AF is 1.5% up to 60 years of age, and 8% at 90 years of age.

Warfarin or not?

Many trials have shown that warfarin is superior to aspirin in reducing thromboembolism in non-rheumatic AF by up to 68% (compared with 28%). However, these studies are generally based on patients in secondary care with higher risks, and the selected/excluded patient groups have been quite strict and then well monitored. Most of the studies compared either aspirin or warfarin with placebo, not with each other.

○ (1999) Primary prevention of arterial thromboembolism in non-rheumatic AF in primary care: RCT comparing two intensities of coumarin with aspirin. *BMJ.* **319**: 958–64.
In this primary care study of 729 patients aged over 60 years, neither low- nor standard-intensity anticoagulation was found to be better than aspirin.

○ (2001) Meta-analysis of anti-coagulation/aspirin in non-rheumatic AF: 5 RCTs from the past 12 years. *BMJ.* **322**: 321–6.
This study found no significant difference in cardiovascular events, although there was a higher risk of bleeds in the warfarin group. Needless to say, some people are disputing this review, which highlights the continued lack of consensus.

○ (2001) *Br J Gen Pract.* **51**: 884–90.
This recent UK study showed that up to 60% of patients with AF have contraindications for either warfarin or aspirin. When deciding on appropriate treatment in the 40% of patients who are eligible, it is important to discuss the risks vs. the benefits.

○ (2001) *Eur Heart J.* **22**: 1852–923 (or www.eurheartj.com).
The European Society of Cardiology, the American Heart Association and the American College of Cardiology have released a 71-page document on the management of AF.

○ (2002) Screening to identify undiagnosed patients. Randomised trial of two approaches to screening for AF in UK general practice. *Br J Gen Pract.* **52**: 373–80.
This study concludes that nurse-led screening for AF in general practice is feasible and effective in identifying a substantial number of patients who could benefit from antithrombotic therapy.

Smoking

- Smoking is the number-one preventable cause of ill health (120 000 deaths/year).

- One in four adults in the UK smoke (13 million in total in the UK).

- The cost to the NHS is £1500 million/year.

- 70% of smokers want to stop (National Statistics 2000).

- Smoking cessation by someone with angina decreases their chances of having a myocardial infarction by up to 50%.

○ (1982) *Am J Epidemiol.* **115**: 231.

1998 White Paper

In this framework for the NHS on smoking cessation, funding was only guaranteed in new Health Action Zones.

It was recommended that practitioners should:

- assess smoking 'at every opportunity'!
- advise patients to stop smoking
- provide accurate information
- recommend nicotine replacement therapy (NRT)
- refer patients to specialist services as necessary
- follow up patients.

February 2000 Royal College of Physicians initiative on 'Nicotine Addiction in Britain'

- Government should provide access to evidence-based smoking cessation services.
- NRT is effective and should be available by NHS prescription.
- It is recommended that GPs should give brief advice at least once a year, and if there is a positive response they should refer the patient to a QUIT clinic (or local equivalent).

Intervention	Success rate at 1 year
Brief opportunistic advice from GPs	2%
Face-to-face behavioural support from specialist	7%
Nicotine gum	5%
Zyban (300 mg/day)	9%
Behavioural support in clinic with NRT or Zyban	13–19%

Coronary Heart Disease National Service Framework, March 2000

- NHS and partner agencies should contribute to a reduction in the prevalence of smoking in the local population.
- Advice about how to stop smoking, including the use of NRT, is highlighted as a priority in people with diagnosed CHD or other occlusive arterial disease.
- In secondary prevention, annual clinical audit should look at recorded smoking status and, for smokers, the delivery of or referral for appropriate advice.

Monitoring Trends and Determinants in Cardiovascular Disease (MONICA)

o (2000) *Lancet*. **355**: 668–9.
This epidemiological WHO study monitored 100 000 men and women aged 35–64 years from 21 countries over a period of 10 years. The most effective intervention for reducing CHD was stopping smoking (50% risk reduction over 2 years).

Smoking Cessation Action in Primary Care Taskforce (SCAPE), launched in September 2001

• The aim of this initiative was to encourage GPs and practice nurses to maintain the impetus of smoking cessation services.

• It adopts the 30-second approach.
   – Do you smoke?
   – Would you like to stop?
   – Would you like my help with stopping?

• A major concern of GPs (in a survey published by SCAPE in May 2001) is workload implications.

• With regard to smoking cessation services, 93% of GPs thought this was 'the best thing you could do for their health'.

• Around 91% of GPs delay advising patients to stop because of time pressures.

• There have been many published papers looking at ways to encourage patients to stop smoking (including several Cochrane Reviews).

o (2003) Predictors of long-term outcome of a smoking cessation programme in primary care. *Br J Gen Pract*. **53**: 101–7.
This study showed that the probability of smoking cessation can be predicted. Willingness to participate, increasing age and previous attempts to stop were all positive predictors.

o (2000) *Br J Gen Pract*. **50**: 207–10.
This qualitative study concluded that GPs should make greater use of problem-orientated opportunities to discuss smoking (i.e. when patients present with a smoking-related problem).

o (1999) Should smoking cessation cost a packet? *Br J Gen Pract*. **49**: 127–80.
This does *not* support the view that free NRT gives better results than that bought by the patient.

o (1997) *NEJM*. **337**: 1195–202 and (1999) *NEJM*. **340**: 685–91.
These two randomised controlled trials support the view that bupropion improves a person's chances of quitting, if used together with regular counselling sessions.

Given recent adverse publicity (presumably), the apparent demand for Zyban has decreased. Bupropion is known to lower the seizure threshold so should not be prescribed with certain drugs, e.g. antidepressants, antipsychotics, tramadol, theophyllines (check your *British National Formulary*). Similarly, it should not be prescribed to people at risk of seizures or to diabetics (owing to the risk of hypoglycaemia).

○ (2001) Qualitative study of pilot payment aimed at increasing GPs' anti-smoking advice to smokers. *BMJ*. **323**: 432–5.
GPs and practice nurses were negative about this new health promotion despite payment, as the latter does not automatically generate effective activity.
  GPs felt that the payment was insufficient to reflect the work needed to identify patients.

○ (2001) Intervention study to evaluate pilot health promotion payment aimed at increasing GPs' anti-smoking advice to smokers. *BMJ*. **323**: 435–6.
Since the 1990s the Government has tried to influence health promotion activity by GPs through payment schemes. It was found that the pilot payments did not change GPs' or nurses' behaviour with regard to advising patients to stop smoking.

○ (2001) *Arch Gen Psychiatry*. **58**: 821–7.
The brains of long-term smokers were found to show neurochemical abnormalities similar to those found in animals treated with antidepressants. This suggests the hypothesis that smoking has antidepressant properties.

NICE (National Institute for Clinical Excellence) guidelines on smoking cessation

• NRT and bupropion are recommended for smokers who want to quit.

• They should only be prescribed if a quit date has been set.

• The initial prescription should ideally last for 2 weeks after the quit date and only be continued if the patient is still trying to quit.

• If the patient does not stop, another course should not be prescribed for 6 months.

Miscellaneous

Cardiac rehabilitation

The aim is to restore the patient to the best possible function after myocardial infarction and minimise the risk of recurrence.

British Heart Foundation Factfile September 2000
Cardiac rehabilitation improves risk, morbidity, mortality and psychosocial outcome. However, it needs to be an individual programme rather than prescriptive, and must have a multidisciplinary approach. Several studies have shown that the programmes are cost-effective (both medically and socially).
  The National Service Framework for CHD recommends cardiac rehabilitation as part of secondary prevention within the NHS trust.

○ (1989) An overview of randomised clinical trials of rehabilitation with exercise after MI. *Circulation*. **80**: 234–44.
This showed a reduction in cardiac mortality of 20–25%.

Homocysteine

- In 2002, the British Cardiac Society presented research data showing that elevated homocysteine levels (>12 mmol/L) doubled the risk of a second coronary event.

- High homocysteine levels in the general population are mainly due to inadequate folate and vitamin B concentrations.

- There is not enough evidence to recommend that homocysteine levels be used as part of the routine CHD risk assessment.

- Guidelines from the International Atherosclerosis Society recommend screening homocysteine levels in high-risk patients (not agreed by the National Screening Committee). If the levels are checked and found to be raised, treatment with diet or 400 µg folic acid should be initiated and the test repeated after 3 months. If the levels are still raised, higher doses of folate, vitamin B_6 and vitamin B_{12} are advocated.

C-reactive protein (CRP)

A CRP concentration of >3 mg/L may indicate the need for intensive treatment to reduce the cardiovascular risk. US guidelines suggest case selection and use for patients with a 10-year CHD risk of 10–20%.

Gastrointestinal tract

Upper gastrointestinal disorders

Dyspepsia

This is defined as 'chronic or recurrent pain or discomfort centred in the upper abdomen'.

○ (1991) *Gastroenterol Int.* **4**: 145–60.

- Around 40% of the population complain of dyspepsia, and 25% consult their GP.

- Around 25% of patients with dyspepsia will have *Helicobacter pylori*.

- The NHS spends more than £1 billion/year managing dyspepsia, and more than 50% of this is on drugs.

- Causes:
  60%: non-ulcer/functional dyspepsia
  40%: gastro-oesophageal reflux disorder (GORD), duodenal and gastric ulcer disease, gastric cancer.

- ALARM symptoms (**A**naemia, weight **L**oss, **A**norexia, **R**efractory problems, **M**elaena or Swallowing problems) should be referred for urgent investigation.

Helicobacter pylori

This affects 20% of people under 40 years of age and 50% of people over 60 years.

H. pylori is a Gram-negative bacterium that colonises the stomach. Its exact role in peptic ulceration (and coronary heart disease) is unclear. It can affect the stomach in childhood, causing chronic gastritis which can lead to peptic ulcer disease. The rate of infection is lower with higher socio-economic class, so it is thought to be related to overcrowding.

○ (2000) *Lancet*. **355**: 358–62.

Reinfection in adults is rare, so eradication treatment is almost curative.

Disease associations (not exhaustive!) include: duodenal ulcer (95%), gastric ulcer (60–70%), and gastric cancer (60%). GORD shows no association, and eradication may make symptoms worse.

Maastricht-2 states that all patients on long-term non-steroidal anti-inflammatory drugs (NSAIDs) should be tested for *H. pylori*.

Management

In cases of confirmed ulcers, eradication speeds healing and reduces recurrence (NNT = 2). This is not the case in GORD (NNT = 17). Most guidelines suggest that it is not necessary to test for *H. pylori* if there is a known duodenal ulcer, but to treat empirically and investigate if ALARM symptoms occur or they do not improve.

○ (2000) *BMJ*. **321**: 659–64 and (1999) *BMJ*. **319**: 1040–4.
  These meta-analyses of patients with *H. pylori* associated with non-ulcer dyspepsia showed an improvement in symptoms if *H. pylori* was eradicated. There are obviously trials that dispute this.

A triple regimen is more successful than the double. There is no difference between the different triple regimens, and 1 week is as successful as 2 weeks of treatment.

One randomised controlled trial in patients with GORD came to the conclusion that eradication was neither beneficial nor harmful, and 25% of patients still had symptoms after successful eradication.

Long-term treatment with NSAIDs

○ (2002) *Gut*. **51**: 329–35.
  This Swiss study recently advocated a test-and-treat policy for people who require long-term NSAIDS. The randomised controlled trial found that if *H. pylori*-positive patients had eradication therapy for *H. pylori* while taking NSAIDs, there was a 1% incidence of ulcer. This increased to 6% in those who were untreated.

Non-invasive tests for H. pylori

1 *Serology*. This does not distinguish between old and active infection (IgG anti-bodies can remain in the circulation for up to 9 months after eradication) (i.e. 50% of positives could be false negatives). At present this is a suboptimal test and not recommended. Its sensitivity is 60–85% and its specificity is 80%, depending on which paper you read.

2 *Urea breath test*. Urea is hydrolysed by *H. pylori* urease, which converts it to carbon dioxide and ammonia. The specificity and sensitivity are 95%, and this is thought to be the best test at present. It is easy to use in primary care (but does still have to be sent to the lab for analysis). It should not be used while the patient is taking antacids/proton-pump inhibitors, because of the risk of false-negative results.

   The test becomes negative once *H. pylori* is eradicated. It is more expensive than serology but reduces the need for endoscopy, so is more cost-effective in the long run.

   ○ (2002) *BMJ*. **324**: 999–1002.
      This study concluded that this test should be the preferred method.

3 *Stool antigen detection test*. The specificity and sensitivity are 90%, but you need a lot of the good stuff! It is not known whether positive tests should ultimately lead to endoscopy (other than with serology testing).

   ○ (1999) *Gut*. **45**: 186–90.
      This paper looked at patients ⩽45 years of age who were HLO-positive on breath test and rando-mised them to empirical treatment or endoscopy. These arms had similar clinical outcomes and could potentially save 73% of endoscopies. No conclusion was reached about eradication in non-ulcer dyspepsia.

   ○ (2001) *BMJ*. **322**: 898–901.
      This randomised controlled trial of *H. pylori* testing and endoscopy for dyspepsia in primary care concluded that the cost of both investigations was not offset by the improvement in symptom relief or quality of life.

Invasive test/endoscopy

Histology has a sensitivity and specificity of >90%.

Although it is more invasive and expensive, it is preferable to empirical treatment. It decreases drug consumption, number of visits to the doctor, and sick leave for 2 years after endoscopy compared with the year before, and patients are generally more satisfied with the treatment. The symptomatic outcome (endoscopy vs. empirical treatment) is similar in the two groups.

Role of proton-pump inhibitors (PPIs)

The single-agent approach whereby all dyspeptic symptoms are treated with PPIs regardless of severity is inappropriate. In gastro-oesophageal reflux disorder and non-ulcer dyspepsia, use a step-up or step-down approach. It is inadvisable to use PPIs in any patient with ALARM symptoms.

NICE guidelines suggest a healing dose of PPI until the symptoms improve if there is known ulcer disease. If the symptoms persist, use the lowest dose and least expensive PPI. If NSAIDs are absolutely necessary (i.e. if an ulcer is present), use with a PPI.

Prolonged PPI use can increase the risk of atrophic gastritis if the patient is *H. pylori*-positive.

Antisecretory therapy, especially with PPIs, can mask, obscure and delay endoscopic diagnosis of gastric adenocarcinoma.

○ Bramble *et al.* (2000) *Gut.* **46**: 464–7.

Colorectal cancer

In terms of diagnosis and screening, this 'hot topic' has been around for at least 5 years and will continue to generate interest as pilot studies for *population screening* have been successful, and work is underway to determine how a national screening programme should be implemented. Remember that there is already colonoscopy surveillance in cases of familial adenomatous polyposis (if genetic tests are positive after 15 years of age) and for patients with inflammatory bowel disease.

• Colorectal cancer is the third most common cancer in the UK.

• It kills *c.* 16 000 people every year.

• Around 5% of people with bowel cancer have more than one cancer.

Role of the GP

• Identify high-risk patients – early detection improves 5-year survival.

• Provide detailed counselling and information about the causes of colorectal cancer.

○ Rhodes (2000) *Gut.* **46**: 746–8.
    Around 90% of cases are diet related (high fat and meat intake) and 10% are genetic.

Role of NSAIDs

Several cohort and case-control studies have consistently shown dose-related reductions of colorectal cancer in regular users of these drugs.

There has been only one randomised controlled trial with a 5-year follow-up which showed no benefit. It was postulated that the follow-up was too short and that 10–20 years would be needed to show any effect. The use of aspirin as a chemoprotective agent is not yet advocated for the general population.

Screening tools for bowel cancer

It is estimated that a 10-year screening programme would prevent 5000 new cases and 3000 deaths a year in the UK. Faecal occult blood screening and flexible sigmoidoscopies are the two main screening options.

Faecal occult blood (FOB) screening (Cochrane Review 1998)

- Low sensitivity and specificity (tumour needs to be bleeding) in the range 50–60%.
- Most extensively studied screening test for colorectal cancer.
- False positives with red meat and vegetables rich in peroxidase.
- Several large randomised controlled trials have shown that FOB screening is feasible.
- Two studies have shown a reduction in mortality with FOB screening.
- FOB undertaken every 2 years may reduce mortality by 20%.

Flexible sigmoidoscopy

- Can detect 80% of colorectal cancers.
- Many nurses are now trained to perform flexible sigmoidoscopies, so it is more cost-effective.
- Only detects cancers up to the splenic flexure (50% of cancers are proximal).
- A multicentre mortality trial is due for completion in late 2003.

Colonoscopy

- Gold standard but expensive, requires bowel preparation and is more invasive.

Barium enema

- There have been no population screening studies using the barium enema.

DNA stool screening

- Tumour DNA can be detected in stools from an early stage.
- The technique is still in the early stages of development, and therefore although non-invasive is still expensive.
  - ○ (2002) *Lancet*. **359**: 403–4.
    Researchers were able to identify 37% of cancers using a genetic marker specific for the tumour, with no false positives.

Coeliac disease

Only around 20% of patients with coeliac disease are currently being diagnosed.

○ (1999) Banbury Coeliac Study. *BMJ*. **318**: 164–7.
This study was set up to determine the under-diagnosis of coeliac disease and to gain further insight into the way in which it presents in general practice, over a 1-year period. In the study, 1000 patients were tested for endomysial antibody (other antibody tests could include gliadin and reticulin). In total, 30 of these were positive with a positive biopsy result; 15 out of 30 patients presented with anaemia and 25 out of 30 patients presented with non-gastrointestinal symptoms.

○ (2001) Association of adult coeliac disease with IBS: a case-controlled study in patients fulfilling the ROME II criteria referred to secondary care. *Lancet*. **358**: 1504–8.
This study found that irritable bowel syndrome was significantly associated with coeliac disease.

GPs can prescribe gluten-free foods to patients with coeliac disease or dermatitis herpetiformis, but must endorse the prescription 'ACBS' (According to Borderline Substance Act), otherwise the script may be queried. Compliance with a gluten-free diet has been shown to improve with medical follow-up. The British Society for Gastroenterology suggests that this is done yearly.

Long-term complications of coeliac disease include small bowel lymphoma and osteoporosis (up to 50%). The Primary Care Society for Gastroenterology guidelines suggest that a DEXA scan should be performed at the time of diagnosis and repeated after the menopause for women, or at the age of 55 years for men. If a fragility fracture occurs at any age, a scan should be performed.

The Coeliac Society produces an annual list of food products that are gluten-free, which is available to members (www.coeliac.co.uk).

The Department of Health advises prophylactic immunisation against *Pneumococcus* in coeliac disease patients over 2 years of age, due to the risk of hyposplenism.

Mental health

The New Mental Health Act (revised from 1983)

The definition of a mental disorder is 'any disability or disorder of the mind or brain, whether permanent or temporary, which results in an impairment or disturbance of mental functioning'. Not only is the definition broad, but it is an emotive subject on which patients and the public have many preconceived ideas, especially with regard to loss of rights. The reformed act goes some way towards addressing difficult issues, but it is important to remember that there is a distinct difference between treating mental disorders and exercising social control.

The White Paper *Reforming the Mental Health Act* (January 2001) is not yet law, although the aim is to make it so by late 2003, once certain elements have been tested.

A New Mental Health (and Public Protection) Act was first published in 1959, the main issues being that decisions on involuntary treatment for mental disorders should become primarily a matter for doctors. In 1983, limits to medical discretion were set out.

The key issues with regard to mental health are listed below.

Risk of patients to themselves and others

- Care and treatment provided should reflect the best interest of the patient.
- Half of the paper is devoted to high-risk patients.
- Perceived failures in community care are the main driving force.

Simpler template for formal assessment

- Assessment will be conducted by two doctors and an approved social worker (no change).
- The template will be set out in a formal care plan which must be of 'direct therapeutic benefit' or address the management of 'behaviours arising from the disorder'.
- After 28 days it will have to be re-authorised by the Mental Health Tribunal (an independent body).
- It will be followed by a care and treatment order applicable in both civil and criminal justice, which will be made by the Mental Health Tribunal or by a court.

Care and treatment in the community

- Care and treatment orders may apply to patients outside hospital.
- There will be contingency plans if patients refuse to take their medication in the community, to prevent such patients becoming a risk to themselves and others.

Safeguards

- There is entitlement to a free legal service.
- There is a statutory obligation for care plans.
- The Mental Health Tribunal is an independent body that takes advice from the clinical team, patients, independent experts and other agencies. It is also concerned with long-term use of compulsory powers. It may exceptionally reserve the right not to accept the clinical supervisor's decision to discharge a patient, if there is serious risk of harm to others.
- The new Commission for Mental Health has responsibilities for maintaining formal powers and looking after people who are subject to care and treatment orders.

○ (2001) Reforming the Mental Health Act. *BMJ*. **322**: 2–3.
  This is a good editorial which looks at some of the issues and touches on aspects that seem to be amiss. It does not address the issues of when a community order should end. It also points out several areas where it is at odds with the National Service Framework for mental health, such as combating discrimination and stigma as well as the fundamental point of developing services that patients will want to use.

○ (1999) *BMJ*. **318**: 549–51 and (1999) *BMJ*. **319**: 1146–7.
  These two papers suggest that mental health services have failed to meet the needs of people with personality disorders, and that the proposed new measures are ethically problematic.

Changing Minds: Every Family in the Land

This is a 5-year campaign organised by Royal College of Psychiatrists to combat the stigmatisation of people with anxiety disorders, severe depression, dementia, schizophrenia, eating disorders, and drug and alcohol dependencies.

Mental Illness: Stigmatisation and Discrimination within the Medical Profession is a report targeted at professionals as part of the above campaign.

In 2001, the World Health Organization published the first global profile of mental health services, which concluded that in most countries mental health is not taken seriously.

Admission under compulsion

This is only to be used if the patient is suffering from a mental disorder and cannot be persuaded to enter hospital voluntarily. Never use it lightly, and always keep comprehensive notes. Acceptance by the receiving hospital is necessary.

Section 2 (assessment)

- This should be used where possible (Section 4 may be more appropriate in general practice).

- The maximum length of stay is 28 days.

- It is applied for by an approved social worker or the patient's nearest relative.

- It is supported by two doctors (one of whom must be Section 12 approved and one of whom has knowledge of the patient). The two doctors must examine the patient within 5 days of each other.

Section 3 (admission and treatment)

- Application is based on two medical recommendations.

- Length of stay is for 6 months initially, typically following on from a Section 2.

Section 4 (emergency in the community)

- The maximum length of stay is 72 hours.

- It is applied for by an approved social worker or the patient's nearest relative.

- It is supported by one doctor, who should have previous knowledge of the patient if possible (both individuals must have seen the patient within 24 hours).

The National Service Framework for Mental Health

- At any one time, one in six adults suffers from a mental illness (mainly anxiety or depression).

- One in 250 people have a psychotic illness (e.g. schizophrenia or bipolar affective disorder).

- Nine in 100 people who consult their GP with a psychiatric problem will be referred to specialist services.

- Mental health is one of four target areas in *Saving Lives: Our Healthier Nation* and there is a specific target to reduce suicide by 20% by 2010.

- The NSF fleshes out policies in the White Paper *Modernising Mental Health Services*.

- An investment in mental health services of £700 million is planned over the next three years.

The NSF has five main areas and seven standards.

Mental health promotion (standard 1)

1 Health and social services should:
    - promote mental health for all
    - combat discrimination against individual groups.

Primary care and access to services (standards 2 and 3)

2 Any service user who contacts their primary healthcare team with a common mental health problem should:
    - have their mental health needs identified and assessed
    - be offered effective treatments and referral if required.

3 Any individual with a common mental health problem should:
    - be able to have 24-hour contact with social services
    - be able to use NHS Direct for first-level advice.

Effective services for people with severe mental illness (standards 4 and 5)

4 All mental health service users on a care programme should:
  - receive care which prevents or anticipates crises and reduces risk
  - have written care plans that include action to be taken in a crisis, as well as GP advice if the patient needs additional help, and that are regularly reviewed by the core co-ordinator
  - be able to access services 24 hours a day 365 days a year.

5 Each service user who is assessed as requiring a period of care away from their home should:
  - have access to an appropriate bed
  - be placed as close to home as possible
  - receive a copy of a written aftercare plan on discharge.

Caring about carers (standard 6)

6 All individuals who provide regular and substantial care for a person on a care programme should:
  - have an annual assessment of their physical and mental needs
  - have their own written care plan.

Preventing suicide (standard 7)

7 All standards 1 to 6, and in addition:
  - supporting local prison staff in preventing suicide among prisoners
  - ensuring the competence of staff
  - developing local systems for suicide audit.

The overall performance will be assessed at national and local level in a number of ways:

- long-term improvement in psychological health of the population, as measured by the National Psychiatric Morbidity Survey

- reduction in suicide rates

- prescribing data

- access to psychiatric services and therapies

- experience of users

- reduction in the number of emergency admissions.

General opinions on the NSF

○ (2001) *BMJ*. **322**: 443.

- It is about time!

- It is workable and clearly set out.

- On the whole, there is an evidence base (but how can you audit discrimination?).

- Investment is planned, but it is never enough.

- It will need a huge drive on staff recruitment, training and support.

- Patients and carers are referred to as 'service users' – interesting!

- It ultimately relies on 24-hour access through NHS Direct, but is this really the best access point for this kind of patient?

- Physical health needs are only highlighted with reference to the carers. We know that patients with severe mental illness have high rates of physical illness, which is often undetected, with twice the mortality of the general population.

○ (2002) *BMJ*. **324**: 61–2. (Further *BMJ* Editorial.)

- It only covers adults up to 65 years of age (cf. discrimination issues). Elderly and young people/children will be addressed in separate service development programmes.

- It supports regional mental health development.

- Plans have been developed by region.

- Implementation team support.

- Bipolar affective disorder has been left out in the cold.

- Facilitators are in place to:
  - form a relationship with the primary healthcare team
  - encourage assessment of current practice
  - offer resources to assist the process of change (e.g. guidelines)
  - promote teamwork and improve links
  - organise educational activity.

○ (2000) *Br J Gen Pract*. **50**: 626.
Interestingly, although facilitators have been shown to improve GP management in cerebrovascular accidents, heart disease and asthma, a randomised controlled trial of six practices with facilitators and six controls has shown that, although recognition of mental illness was improved, there was no change in treatment or outcome. Debate at your leisure!

○ (2001) Dying for a drink. *BMJ*. **323**: 817–18.
In this national confidential enquiry, 40% of people who committed suicide in England and Wales (who had been in contact with the NHS within 1 year of their death) had a history of alcohol misuse, and 19% also misused drugs.
   This is a fundamental area to be targeted if we are to achieve the aims of standard 7.

Suicide Prevention Strategy for England

www.doh.gov.org.uk/mentalhealth/exe-sum-intro.htm
www.nimhe.org.uk

- Around 5000 people take their own life each year.

- Suicide is the commonest cause of death in men under 35 years of age.

- Risk factors include the following:
  - male
  - living alone
  - being unemployed
  - alcohol and drug misuse
  - mental illness.

The strategy was written to support the target set by the White Paper *Saving Lives: Our Healthier Nation* and the NSF for mental health.
   The aim is to reduce death from suicide by at least 20% by 2010.
   The goals of the programme are as follows:

- to reduce the risk to key high-risk groups

- to promote mental well-being in the wider population

- to reduce the availability and lethality of suicide methods

- to improve reporting of suicide behaviour in the media

- to promote research on suicide prevention

- to improve monitoring of progress.

Anyone who self-harms and requires admission should have a follow-up visit by community mental health teams within 1 week. They should not be issued with repeat medication lasting for more than 2 weeks.
   Implementation of the strategy will be the responsibility of the National Institute for Mental Health in England.

Depression

- One in 20 people have clinical depression.

- Around 50% of depression is not diagnosed.

Depression can be a disabling condition, and it is important to be aware of the symptoms and how the many faces of depression can touch every aspect of a person's life. GPs' diagnoses of depression show high levels of concordance with DSM-IV. However, we do still miss up to 50% of cases. This can be improved by a change in consultation style (asking open questions, making eye contact, not inter-rupting, etc.).

○   (2000) *Br J Gen Pract.* **50**: 284.

DSM-IV diagnostic scale

Five of the following symptoms should be present over a 2-week period for the diagnosis of major depression.

Depressed mood or irritability   } at least one of these symptoms
Loss of interest or pleasure

Appetite or weight loss
Sleep loss/change in sleep pattern
Psychomotor agitation or retardation
Fatigue/loss of energy   three or four of these symptoms
Feelings of worthlessness or guilt   to make a total of five
Poor concentration
Recurrent suicidal thoughts/thoughts of death

The above criteria are useful for differentiating between low mood and clinical depression. In chronic depressive illness (dysthymia), be aware that patients may not meet DSM-IV criteria but could still benefit from drug treatment in the short term.

Screening questionnaires

These are useful to aid diagnosis and monitor progress.

● *General Health Questionnaire* – designed for adults, it assesses inability to function normally.

● *Geriatric Depression Scale* (*see below*) – designed for elderly people, it avoids somatic items.

● *Beck Depression Inventory* – designed for patients with more severe depression, it tackles suicidal thinking.

● *Edinburgh Postnatal Depression Scale* – more sensitive than other scales in postna-tal women.

● *Abbreviated Mental Test Score* (*see below*) – it can be used as a guide to dementia.

● *Hamilton Depression Rating Scale* – not ideal for older people, as it includes a number of somatic items that may be positive in older people who are not depressed.

There has been much debate and work on improving the diagnosis of depression in general practice. The Hampshire Depression Project looked at the effect of clinical practice guidelines and practice-based education on the detection and outcome of depression in primary care. They found that there was no improvement in detection when compared with usual care with no extra education/protocols. Needless to say, GPs were criticised for not following guidelines.

○ (2000) *Lancet.* **355**: 185–91.

The Defeat Depression Campaign was run by the Royal College of Psychiatrists and the Royal College of General Practitioners from 1992 to 1996, and was aimed at educating GPs in the recognition and management of depression, as well as enhancing public awareness.

Abbreviated Mental Test Score (AMTS)

1	Age	0/1
2	Time (to nearest hour)	0/1
3	Address for recall at end – 42 West Street	0/1
4	Year	0/1
5	Name of place (where test was conducted)	0/1
6	Recognition of two people	0/1
7	Date of birth	0/1
8	Year of World War Two	0/1
9	Name of present monarch	0/1
10	Count backwards from 20 to 1	0/1

Geriatric Depression Scale (GDS)

1	Are you basically satisfied with your life?	Yes/**No**
2	Have you dropped many of your activities or interests?	**Yes**/No
3	Do you feel that your life is empty?	**Yes**/No
4	Do you often get bored?	**Yes**/No
5	Are you in good spirits most of the time?	Yes/**No**
6	Are you afraid that something bad is going to happen to you?	**Yes**/No
7	Do you feel happy most of the time?	Yes/**No**
8	Do you feel helpless?	**Yes**/No
9	Do you prefer to stay at home rather than going out and doing new things?	**Yes**/No
10.	Do you feel that you have more problems with memory than most?	**Yes**/No
11	Do you think it is wonderful to be alive now?	Yes/**No**
12	Do you feel pretty worthless the way you are now?	**Yes**/No
13	Do you feel full of energy?	Yes/**No**
14	Do you feel your situation is hopeless?	**Yes**/No
15	Do you think that most people are better off than you are?	**Yes**/No

Scoring: Answers indicating depression are highlighted in bold type. Each scores 1 point. This scoring guidance should not be seen by the patient. A score of ≫5 indicates probable depression.

Drug treatment in depression

You need to ask yourself what you are trying to achieve:

- *improvement* in mood, social and occupational function, quality of life
- *reduction* in morbidity and mortality
- *prevention* of a recurrence
- *minimisation* of adverse effects of treatment.

Antidepressants

Systematic reviews have shown that there is no clinically significant difference in effectiveness between different classes of drugs. All of them produce an improvement of 50–60%. On average, people on selective serotonin reuptake inhibitors (SSRIs) are less likely to stop treatment because of side-effects, but this amounts to only small differences in numbers, which are not thought to be enough to justify choosing SSRIs as a first-line treatment. The side-effect profiles of different drugs mean that some will be used to better effect in the treatment of depression with certain coexistent symptoms. It is important to be aware of potential drug interactions.

SSRIs vs. tricyclic antidepressants (TCAs) (Clinical Evidence 2000)
Three randomised controlled trials showed no difference in overall effectiveness.

- ○ (2000) *J Affect Dis.* **58**: 19–36 and (1998) *J Affect Dis.* **48**: 125–33.
- ○ (2000) *Am J Med.* **108**: 54–64.

SSRIs are 30 times more expensive than TCAs.
   If there are no side-effects, the drug should be used for 6 weeks before changing class. When stopping the drug, tail it off over 4 weeks.

- ○ (2001) Inhibition of serotonin reuptake by antidepressants and upper gastrointestinal bleeding in elderly patients: retrospective cohort study. *BMJ.* **323**: 655–8.
  This study showed an increased risk of gastrointestinal bleeding in elderly patients on antidepressants which inhibit serotonin reuptake. When controlled for age, the risk of gastrointestinal bleeding increased by 10.7%.
- ○ (2002) Meta-analysis of effects and side-effects of low-dose TCA in depression. *BMJ.* **325**: 991–5.
  This study concluded that treatment with low-dose TCA was justified and that there was better compliance with this regime.

St John's wort (Hypericum perforatum)
This is a low-grade monoamine oxidase inhibitor which is widely dispensed over the counter for low mood and depression. A systematic review of 27 studies (Cochrane Library, 1999) concluded that it was more effective than placebo. However, various different preparations of *Hypericum* were used in each study.

o (1999) *Hypericum* extract vs. imipramine or placebo in patients with moderate depression: randomised multi-centre study for 8 weeks. *BMJ.* **319**: 1534–9.
   This study found that *Hypericum* 350 mg three times a day was at least as effective as imipramine, and both were more effective than placebo.

o (2000) Comparison of St John's wort and imipramine for treating depression: randomised controlled trial. *BMJ.* **321**: 536–9.
   This study showed that *Hypericum* was therapeutically equivalent to imipramine, but had a better side-effect profile. A total of 157 patients were scored on the Hamilton Depression Scale.

It is worth noting that *Hypericum* can induce liver enzymes and may interact with digoxin, theophylline, warfarin and the combined oral contraceptive pill (consult the *British National Formulary*!). Different *Hypericum* products also vary widely in composition.

Non-drug treatments (*Evidence-based Medicine*, 2000)

Cognitive behavioural therapy (CBT)
This is a structured treatment aimed at changing the dysfunctional beliefs and negative automatic thoughts that characterise depressive disorders. This form of treatment requires the therapist to have a high level of training.

   The simple understanding is that CBT and problem solving are successful, whereas counselling is less so, although it does result in a high level of patient satisfaction. More recent studies looking at the long-term outcome have on the whole found no difference between groups.

o (2002) Managing depression as chronic disease: a randomised trial of ongoing treatment in primary care. *BMJ.* **325**: 934–7.
   This study showed that there was no significant difference between the two groups (1-year drug treatment vs. 6-session CBT). More people would opt for CBT than for drug treatment, and this group did better than if they were randomly allocated to it, implying that patients should be allowed to choose between the treatments. However, there were four arms to the trial, so the numbers were relatively small. Moreover, the 12-month follow-up was poor.

o (2001) *BMJ.*
   This study found that ongoing intervention over a period of 2 years improved symptoms and remission rates and increased average rates of antidepressant use. Remission rates increased by 33% (95% CI, 7–46) with the enhanced care.

The future

Urinary screening may allow neurochemical profiling of depression subtypes, enabling more rational prescribing of antidepressants.

Schizophrenia

The first description of schizophrenia appeared in the eighteenth century. It has a 1% lifetime prevalence, with 25% of patients being cared for by their GP. The diagnosis is made on the basis of the WHO International Classification of Disease (ICD-10), which looks for clear evidence of past or present psychosis, absence of prominent affective symptoms and a minimum duration of illness. We also need to look for negative symptoms such as blunted affect or poor motivation.

Schneider's first-rank symptoms can be summarised as follows:

- auditory hallucinations

- thought withdrawal or insertion

- thought broadcasting

- somatic passivity

- feelings or actions that are perceived as being under external control

- delusional perceptions.

How to manage a first episode of schizophrenia

- The early stages of the disease form can predict the course and outcome of the illness.

- Early treatment may result in a better prognosis and functional outcome. This is not as easy as it sounds, given the insidious nature of the condition as well as the reluctance to make such an early diagnosis.

- Around 70% of people will relapse within 5 years after the first attack. Therefore early withdrawal of treatment is not recommended.

- Effective treatment consists of the following:
  - a multidisciplinary team
  - drugs to control symptoms (no specific recommendations)
  - 'intensive' community rehabilitation ⎫ improve long-term
  - family therapy   ⎬ social functioning
  - psychological work (e.g. CBT)   ⎭ after the acute phase

○ (2000) *BMJ*. **321**: 522.

The new atypicals/antipsychotics

○ (1999) *Schizophr Res*. **35**: 51–68.

There is substantial evidence that these drugs achieve good results with the positive symptoms. Even so, up to 30% of patients do not respond to psychopharmacology, and negative symptoms are even less responsive. There is some evidence that the new antipsychotics reduce the rate of relapse during maintenance treatment.

The side-effect profile seems to be better, with fewer extrapyramidal side-effects. Note that clozapine decreases the white cell count and the latter therefore needs to be monitored.

The new antipsychotics should be considered as first-line treatment in newly diagnosed cases, where there has been no response to first-line therapy or where extrapyramidal side-effects have been a problem. Non-compliance is a complex issue, but the new dissolve-in-the-mouth tablet addresses this. These drugs are insoluble in oil, so are unlikely to be available as a depot formulation.

○ (1999) *BMJ.* **319**: 1045–8.

Prevention of schizophrenia

Yale University is recruiting people with a strong family history of schizophrenia or who show early signs of psychotic behaviour, in order to look at the effects of olanzapine. Oxford University attempted a similar study some years ago, but had difficulty in recruiting and allocating groups because of lack of understanding of the predictive power of clinical signs.

Brief summary of NICE schizophrenia guidelines, December 2002

The guidelines are relevant to adults over 18 years of age and to those diagnosed with schizophrenia below the age of 60 years. There are three phases.

1 Initiation of treatment (first episode):
   - early referral to secondary care and involvement of other services
   - early treatment – suggest discussion with psychiatrist and urgent referral
   - consider atypicals (e.g. olanzapine) as first-line treatment.

2 Treatment of acute episode:
   - single drug – administer at *BNF* dose range for a minimum of 6 weeks, and monitor the response
   - may need rapid tranquillisation
   - be aware of side-effects (e.g. risk of diabetes and weight gain with some atypicals)
   - address other needs (psychological, social, occupational, etc.)
   - high risk of relapse – if you are treating a relapse, you need to continue treatment for 1–2 years
   - slow withdrawal of treatment and monitor for 2 years after last acute episode.

3 Promoting recovery (primary care):
   - care register (essential)
   - monitor mental health and treatment alongside secondary care
   - consider referral in the following circumstances:
     - problem with compliance
     - poor response to treatment
     - suspected comorbid substance misuse
     - increased risk to self or others
     - new to practice list – for assessment and care programme
     - service user prefers not to receive care from GP.

Rapid tranquillisation

- If an intramuscular preparation is required, give lorazepam and/or haloperidol. If haloperidol is used, anticholinergics should be administered to reduce the risk of dystonia and extra pyramidal side-effects.

- Flumazenil must be available.

- If used, make sure you know the following procedures: cardiopulmonary resuscitation (CPR), nursing in the recovery position, blood pressure and pulse monitoring. Following the event, the patient should be able to discuss and write their version of events in the notes.

- CPR skills certification should be updated annually.

Document everything clearly.

The following are essential across all phases:

- optimism
- getting help early
- assessment
- working in partnership
- consent
- accurate information
- addressing language and culture
- addressing the issue of advance directives (although limited in schizophrenia).

Eating disorders

The lifetime prevalence of eating disorders in young women is as follows (note that there is an even social class distribution):

- anorexia nervosa: 0.5–3.7%
- bulimia nervosa: 1.1–4.2%.

Up to 20% will die as a result of their illness.
    Many people do not ask for help, so as GPs we can play a vital role in detection of these disorders. Recognised risk factors include genetic factors (we do not know what is inherited – possibly a vulnerable personality type), cultural values, childhood obesity, early onset of puberty, adverse life experiences, extreme shyness, bullying, family functional style and low self-esteem.

○ (2000) *Br J Gen Pract.* **50**: 21.
   A lot of clues boil down to personality traits which were looked at in this paper.

○ American Psychiatric Association (1994)
   In diagnosis, if diagnostic criteria for both bulimia and anorexia are met, the diagnosis of anorexia takes precedence.

Early diagnosis and intervention give a better outcome. Cognitive behavioural therapy and SSRIs have both been shown to improve short-term outcome compared with placebo, but it is not yet clear whether remission rates are reduced (Cochrane Library).

Standards 2 and 3 of the National Service Framework for mental health outline the need to improve healthcare for patients with anorexia nervosa and bulimia nervosa.

SCOFF questionnaire

○ (1999) *BMJ.* **319**: 1467–8.
   This questionnaire was designed at St George's Hospital, London by Dr J Morgan and colleagues in order to give specialists a simple screening tool with which to identify eating disorders. It consists of five questions, and one point is scored for each 'Yes' answer. A score of >2 indicates a likely problem.

• Do you make yourself **S**ick because you feel uncomfortably full?

• Do you worry that you have lost **C**ontrol over how much you eat?

• Have you recently lost more than **O**ne stone in a three-month period?

• Do you believe yourself to be **F**at when others say you are too thin?

• Would you say that **F**ood dominates your life?

The researchers compared this tool with more lengthy questionnaires and obtained excellent results of 100% sensitivity and 87.5% specificity (12.5% false-positive rate).

○ (2002) The SCOFF questionnaire and clinical interview for eating disorders in general practice: comparative study. *BMJ.* **325**: 755–6.
   This study looked at the use of the SCOFF questionnaire to identify patients in primary care. It detected all women with diagnosed anorexia and bulimia. In summary, it concluded that it was an efficient tool for detecting eating disorders in adults.

Counselling in general practice

Around 51% of general practices have an on-site counsellor.

Counselling is designed to help people work on their problems and become more skilled in helping themselves. It is a disciplined psychological intervention that requires specialist training in the different styles (e.g. directive, informative, confrontational, supportive etc.). There is documented evidence that, if selected appropriately, it is effective. Counsellors have their own professional code of ethics and practice, and they must hold current membership of a professional body (e.g.

the British Association for Counselling and Psychotherapy). Support for each other within the service, in terms of debriefing, is on the whole excellent.

Appropriate referral and assessment are essential for cost-effective intervention. Most counselling consists of 6 to 12 sessions.

Suitable candidates for brief focal counselling include those who:

- are able to express feelings and thoughts

- are able to trust the counsellor

- have mild to moderate difficulties (e.g. depression, relationship problems, anxiety, bereavement, emotional or psychological difficulties)

- are able to bear disturbing or conflicting feelings.

Unsuitable candidates include those who:

- have moderate to severe difficulties (e.g. schizophrenia, dementia, substance abuse, personality disorders, risk of suicide)

- are silent or withdrawn

- are prone to over-intellectualisation

- have no close relationships

- lack ability to think about self.

  ○ (2000) Counselling in general practice. *Drug Ther Bull.* **38**: 49–52.
    There is currently marked regional variation in the UK, which may change in response to primary care groups/trusts and National Service Frameworks. There have been relatively few randomised controlled trials comparing counselling with usual general practice care. However, a meta-analysis of four randomised controlled trials suggests 'statistically better' psychological symptom levels after treatment than if just receiving GP care.

Chronic fatigue syndrome

  ○ (2000) Detailed review of CFS. *BMJ.* **320**: 292–6.

Chronic fatigue syndrome (CFS), also known as myalgic encephalitis (ME) is defined as disabling fatigue associated with other symptoms (e.g. musculoskeletal pain, sleep disturbance, impaired concentration, headaches). The cause is not yet understood. The prevalence is 0.2–2.6% at present.

Treatment with antidepressants may be useful, especially if the condition is associated with depression, insomnia or myalgia.

  ○ (2000) *Am J Med.* **108**: 99–105.
    This study found that a polypeptide involved in the antiviral response was more common in CFS. This may be of help in the future when trying to distinguish the syndrome from depression and other diseases.

Treatment of CFS

Exercise

Several trials have looked at graded exercise programmes.

○ (1997) *BMJ*. **314**: 1647–52.
   This study of 66 people who took part in a 12-week exercise programme building up to 30 minutes showed a significant improvement in symptoms.

○ (1998) *Br J Psychiatry*. **172**: 485–90.
   In this study of 136 people there were four arms to the trial (placebo, exercise, fluoxetine and a combination). Despite the small numbers in each arm, and the fact that some individuals withdrew from the trial, exercise was associated with a significant improvement.

○ (2001) *BMJ*. **322**: 387.
   This study looked at the evidence-based explanation of symptoms and graded exercise with a 1-year follow-up. There was a significantly better outcome (70% vs. 6% for the control) with patient empowerment.

Cognitive behavioural therapy

A systematic review of three randomised controlled trials has found that if CBT is delivered by highly skilled therapists in specialist centres there is a good outcome (Cochrane Library, 1998) over a period of 6–12 months.

○ (2001) *Br J Gen Pract*. **51**: 9.
   This randomised controlled trial of CBT vs. counselling (six sessions of each) found that both were equally effective, with a 50% improvement being obtained at 6 months. In economic terms, counselling would be the better option, given the extra training and time needed with CBT.

Medically unexplained symptoms

○ (2001) *Drug Ther Bull*. **39**: 5.

Around one in five new consultations are by patients with physical symptoms for which there is no organic cause. In a third of cases they persist and can cause distress and disability.

General practice is about dealing with symptoms that do not fit the disease model. Do not make the mistake of labelling symptoms MUS (medically unexplained symptoms) until a thorough clinical assessment and appropriate investigations have been carried out.

It is thought that, although by definition the cause is unknown, these symptoms are due to a complex interaction of biological, psychological, social and cultural factors.

Management

It is important to acknowledge the symptoms and distress, and to provide continuity of care.

Antidepressants

These can be useful, especially if the patient is experiencing pain or difficulty in sleeping, whether or not they are depressed. A benefit is usually seen within 1–7 days (i.e. quickly!). The number needed to treat is 3.

Reattribution

This involves demonstrating an understanding of the patient's complaints by taking a history of related physical, mood and social factors, making the patient feel understood, and making the link between symptoms and psychological problems.

Cognitive behavioural therapy

This has been shown in systematic reviews to be beneficial, particularly in reducing physical symptoms.

○ (2003) Beyond somatisation: a review of the understanding and treatment of medically unexplained physical symptoms. *Br J Gen Pract.* **53**: 233–41.
  This review article looks at the evidence for complex interactions between physical and cognitive processes. It discusses the complex adaptive system, a model which examines internal and external interaction.

Frequent attenders

This is usually a different group of people.
  The average GP attendance per patient is three to four times per year.
  The characteristics of high attenders include the following:

• multiple health problems

• lower social class

• medically unexplained symptoms

• a belief that reattendance is necessary in order to obtain the right treatment.

○ (2001) *Br J Gen Pract.* **51**: 987–94.
  This study showed that psychosocial, lifestyle and health status variables help to predict high GP attendance rates among adults.

Elderly care

National Service Framework for the elderly

This was published in March 2001 (www.doh.gov.uk/nsf/olderpeople.htm).
  It is an action plan to improve health and social services for older people wherever they live. It focuses on the following:

- removing age discrimination

- patient-centred care

- promoting older people's health and independence

- management of specific clinical conditions.

The eight standards are listed below.

1 Root out age discrimination, providing care on the basis of clinical need alone.

2 Person-centred care – treat patients as individuals. There will be a single assessment process with integrated provision of services. GPs will mainly be involved in the contact assessment.

3 Intermediate care – to enable early hospital discharge and to prevent premature or unnecessary admission to long-term residential care.

4 General hospital care – delivered through appropriate specialist care, by staff with the skills to meet their needs.

5 Stroke – the NHS will take action to prevent strokes (both primary and secondary), will provide treatment by specialist stroke services and will offer a multidisciplinary programme of secondary prevention and rehabilitation.

6 Falls – the NHS and councils will take action to prevent falls and reduce resultant fractures or other injuries. Advice will be provided through a specialised falls service.

7 Mental health in older people – there will be access to integrated mental health services (for patients and carers).

8 Promotion of health and active life in older age.

As well as the eight standards listed above, there are five other major projects under way to improve the quality, availability and consistency of services:

- changes in long-term care funding, including the availability of NHS nursing care

- expansion of intermediate care (and community equipment) services

- establishment of Care Direct to provide comprehensive information and ease of access to health, housing, social care and social security

- various initiatives (retirement health check, flu immunisations) to help older people to stay healthy

- use of Section 31 of the Health Act 1999 to promote joint working between the NHS and social services.

Progress will be overseen by the *NHS Modernisation Board* and the *Older People's Taskforce*.

The Department of Health will publish the *Information Strategy for Older People*, describing how GPs will be supported in achieving it.

Falls

- Falls are the leading cause of accidental death in people over 75 years of age, and they result in large costs to the NHS.

- Every year 33–50% of people aged over 65 years suffer a fall, of whom 20% will need medical help and 10% will have sustained a fracture.

One systematic review has suggested that complex interventions which target modification of multiple risk factors on the basis of individual health assessments decreased the number of people who experienced falls.

○ (2000) Guidelines for the prevention of falls in people aged > 65 years. *BMJ.* **321**: 1007–11.
  This study highlighted gaps in the evidence, including economic evaluations. There is a body of evidence advocating multifactorial interventions in reducing falls. Trials have shown that assessment of elderly people presenting in Accident and Emergency after a fall and the use of hip protectors in nursing homes are both effective in reducing morbidity.

○ (2000) Effect of preventative home visits to elderly people in the UK: systematic review. *BMJ.* **320**: 754–8.
  This study found no clear evidence in favour of the effectiveness of preventative home visits to elderly people living in the community.

○ (2001) Promoting health and function in an ageing population. *BMJ.* **322**: 728–9.
  This article reviews the evidence for strategies promoting health and function. It concludes that it is necessary to take into account social, mental, economic and environmental determinants of health in old age. Most health benefits can be gained from regular physical activity of moderate intensity, and substantial gains could be made by promoting health and fitness throughout life.

GPs should:

- review repeat prescriptions

- consider referral for physiotherapy

- consider referral for occupational therapy to reduce home hazards

- consider a joint meeting with the relevant primary healthcare team members for individual cases.

○ (2002) Randomised factorial trial of falls prevention among older people living in their own homes. *BMJ.* **325**: 128–31.
  This Australian study of 1090 people aged over 70 years living at home tested three interventions, namely home hazard management, group-based exercise and vision improvement. Group-based exercise was found to be the most potent single intervention tested. Falls were further reduced by the addition of hazard management and vision improvement.

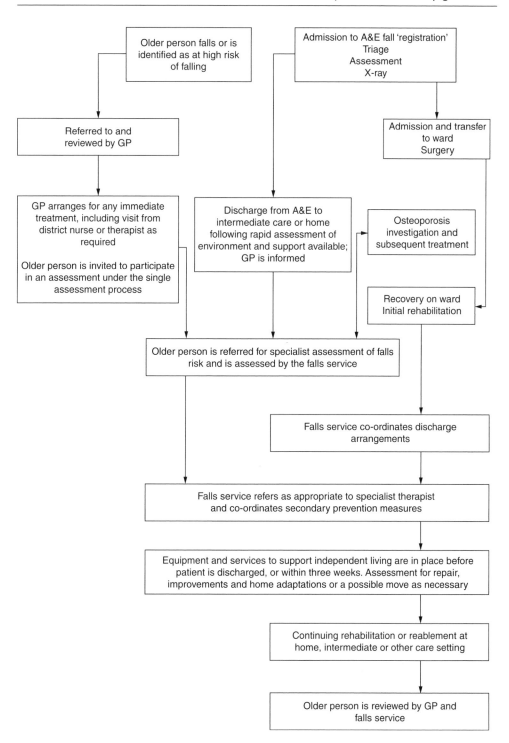

Falls care pathway

o   (2000) Effect of a programme of multifactorial home visits on falls and mobility impairments in elderly peole at risk: rct. *BMJ*. **321**: 994–8.
    This primary care study of 316 people aged over 70 showed that visits had no effect on preventing falls or improving mobility.

Dementia

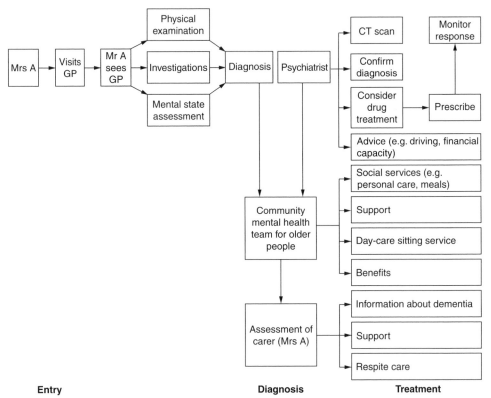

Entry   **Diagnosis**   **Treatment**
Mr A is an 84-year-old former school teacher who is living with his wife. She has arthritis and has begun to worry about her husband's forgetfulness.
The single assessment process could initiate referral to the GP, or the diagnosis itself could initiate an assessment.

NSF flow chart for dementia

Dementia is the chronic deterioration of intellect and personality.

• Around 5% of people over 65 years of age have some form of dementia.

• Around 20% of people over 80 years of age have some form of dementia.

• One in seven elderly people with dementia is in residential care.

• It is important to diagnose dementia early and to identify the type of dementia.

○ (1998) The North of England-based guidelines. *BMJ*. **317**: 802–8.
The key points of these guidelines are centred around accurate diagnosis – investigations, formal cognitive testing, looking for secondary causes, and not forgetting depression.

○ Marshall M (2001) The challenge of looking after people with dementia (editorial). *BMJ*. **323**: 410–11.
The author discusses a paper published in the same issue of the *BMJ* which found that none of the 484 people with dementia living in nursing homes or on hospital wards were experiencing what they refer to as a 'fair standard of care'. The main issues were those of staffing, training and motivation, together with poor-quality buildings.

○ (2000) Are GPs able to accurately diagnose dementia and identify Alzheimer's disease? A comparison with an outpatient memory clinic. *Br J Gen Pract*. **50**: 311–12.
In this cross-sectional study from The Netherlands, GPs were able to assess the firmness of their own dementia diagnoses (i.e. appropriate selection for referral). They were less good at determining the type of dementia.

The Mental Health Foundation has published a report entitled *Tell me the Truth*, which states that most people who develop dementia are not usually told what is wrong with them. It is this information that, although initially difficult to accept, helps patients to understand the changes in themselves and to adapt.

○ (2002) The limited utility of MMSE in screening older people >75 for dementia in primary care. *Br J Gen Pract*. **52**: 1002–3.
The Mini Mental State Examination (MMSE) is recommended as a screening instrument for dementia. A total of 709 subjects completed the MMSE. It was found that the latter had a false-positive rate of 86% for identifying dementia in primary care (202 cases were validated against the GMS-AGECAT diagnostic system) when used with a weighting of 26/30. However, if a cut-off value of 21 was used, the false-positive rate dropped to 59%.

Alzheimer's disease

This is the commonest form of dementia in the UK (accounting for around 60% of cases). There are about 340 000 cases in the UK. In rare cases it is inherited via the AD gene. There are also links to the Apo-E gene, but no useful diagnostic or prognostic test is yet available.

Current management focuses on accurate diagnosis, providing appropriate services, supporting carers and treating non-cognitive problems.

Drugs for Alzheimer's disease
Three cholinesterase inhibitors have been licensed in the UK for mild to moderate Alzheimer's disease, namely donezipil, rivastigmine and galantamine.

They have all been shown to improve cognitive function, global outcome and activities of daily living. There is no convincing evidence that the drugs modify the course of the disease.

○ (2001) *BMJ*. **323**: 123–4.

Summary of NICE guidelines (January 2001) for cholinesterase inhibitors

• Diagnosis must be made by a specialist (according to criteria).

- Activities of daily living, cognition, global and behavioural functioning must be assessed prior to treatment. The MMSE score must be >12.

- Treatment can be continued if there is improvement/no deterioration in the MMSE 2–4 months after reaching the maintenance dose.

- Patients should be reviewed every 6 months.

- Compliance must be ensured.

- GPs may take over prescribing under an agreed shared-care protocol.

It is thought that drug costs may be offset by delaying the need for residential care. Specialist memory clinics/secondary care need to expand (these clinics are recommended in the National Service Framework for older people).

Glutamatergic modulators are a new treatment on the market and are not yet included in the guidelines.

Other treatments

1 *Selegiline and vitamin E*: Treatment with either was found to slow progression of the disease. The Cochrane Review 2000 found that selegiline was more effective than placebo in improving cognitive function, behavioural disturbance and mood.

o (1997) *NEJM*. **336**: 1216–22.

2 *Ginkgo biloba (40 mg three times a day)*: One systematic review of eight randomised controlled trials reported that *Ginkgo biloba* improved cognitive function and was well tolerated by patients with Alzheimer's disease.

o (1999) *Clin Drug Invest*. **17**: 301–8.

3 *Reality orientation*: This involves presenting information designed to reorientate a person in time, place and person. It may be a noticeboard giving the day, date and time, or a member of staff reorientating the patient at each contact. *Clinical Evidence* found one systematic review of small randomised controlled trials that showed an improvement in cognitive function and behaviour compared with no treatment.

Miscellaneous factors

o (2001) Midlife vascular risk factors and Alzheimer's disease in later life: longitudinal population-based study. *BMJ*. **322**: 1447–57.
   This study found that raised systolic blood pressure and high cholesterol levels, especially in combination and in mid-life, increased the risk of Alzheimer's disease in late life. This could have future implications for patient management.

1 *Statins*: A Boston study (yet to be published) is thought to show that statins reduce the risk of developing Alzheimer's disease by up to 80% (the study involved 2581 patients over a period of 5 years).

2 *Hormone replacement therapy*: There is evidence that HRT may be beneficial. One study found that women who had been on HRT for 3 years were 40% less likely to develop Alzheimer's, and for those who had been on it for 10 years the reduction was 60%.

○ (2002) *Lancet*. **288**: 2123–9.

3 *Diet*: Data drawn from PAQUID (a French epidemiological survey) were used, and it was found that people who eat fish or seafood at least once a week were at lower risk of developing dementia, including Alzheimer's disease.

○ (2002) Fish, meat and the risk of dementia: cohort study. *BMJ*. **325**: 923.

4 *Non-steroidal anti-inflammatory drugs*: There is a hypothesis that inflammatory mechanisms play a part in Alzheimer's disease. In one study, 6989 residents of Rotterdam aged over 55 years with no evidence of dementia were included, with a follow-up of 8 years, and the MMSE and Geriatric Mental State Examination were administered. It was found that as NSAID use (other than aspirin) increased, the relative risk of Alzheimer's disease fell from 0.95 to 0.2. The type of NSAID did not influence this effect. No benefit was found in vascular dementia.

○ (2001) NSAIDs and the risk of Alzheimer's disease. *NEJM*. **345**: 515–21.

Detection

○ (2003) Detection of Alzheimer's disease and dementia in the preclinical phase: population-based cohort. *BMJ*. **326**: 245–7.
   This study looked at three tests, namely self-reported memory complaints, a test of global cognitive function and specific cognitive tests. Although only 18% of subjects in the preclinical phase were identified, the test had a positive predictive value of 85–100% for these cases.

Parkinson's disease

The prevalence of Parkinson's disease is one in 1000 at the average age of onset (55 years), and 1 in 200 in those over 65 years of age.

On the whole, treatment is best resisted unless there is functional disability.

○ (2000) *BMJ*. **321**: 1–2.

○ (2000) *Clin Evidence Rev*. **4**: 737.

○ (2000) *NEJM*. **342**: 1484.
   A 5-year randomised controlled trial comparing L-dopa with ropinirole (a D3 receptor agonist) found that ropinirole was better tolerated and patients were less likely to suffer dyskinesias. Large numbers of patients withdrew from both arms of the trial. There is also the rare possibility of sleep occurring as a side-effects of this drug, even in the middle of daily activities.

No drugs have been found to delay progression.

Surgery

Thalamotomy, pallidotomy, deep brain stimulation and foetal nigral implants are all being trialled. The initial results in selected groups have been found to show an improvement in contralateral symptoms of tremor and bradykinesis.

Depression

This is common in Parkinson's disease (up to 50% of cases). It is thought to have neurobiological manifestations rather than being a purely emotional response to the disease.

○ (1999) *J Neurol Neurosurg Psychiatry.* **67**: 492–6.

Guidelines for the management of Parkinson's disease in primary care by the primary care task force for this disorder are available from: Parkinson's Disease, 215 Vauxhall Bridge Road, London SW1 1EJ.

New advances

Gene therapy

○ (2002) *Science.* **298**: 425–9.
    To date this has only been carried out on rats. However, the first human trial has just been approved in the USA.

Dietary supplements

○ (2002) *Arch Neurol.* **59**: 1541–50.
    Co-enzyme Q10 may reduce the functional decline in Parkinson's disease.

Stroke

This is defined as 'sudden loss of neurological function lasting for more than 24 hours'.

- The incidence of stroke is 2 in 1000 (double this in those aged 45–84 years).

- It is the third most common cause of death in the UK and the greatest single cause of disability.

- Around 80% of all strokes are ischaemic.

- Around 50% of patients are physically dependent on others for 6 months after the event.

- The incidence of transient ischaemic attack is 0.4 in 1000 (the future risk of stroke is 10% in the first year and 5% thereafter).

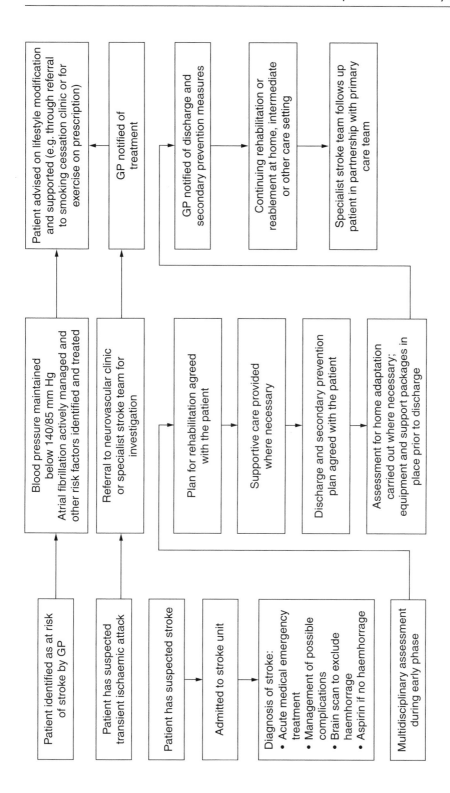

Stroke care pathway

Prevention (primary and secondary)

Hypertension
This accounts for 50% of ischaemic strokes.

British Hypertension Society guidelines state that hypertension persisting for more than 1 month after cerebrovascular accident should be treated. The risk of stroke can be reduced by up to 40% if the diastolic blood pressure is reduced by 6 mmHg or the systolic blood pressure is reduced by 10–12 mmHg (irrespective of whether the blood pressure is elevated or not).

- STOP-2 (Swedish Trial in Older Patients)
  A total of 6614 patients were randomised to beta-blockers and thiazides or ACE inhibitors. Both groups showed a reduction in blood pressure, but there was no major difference in primary end points, including fatal and non-fatal stroke.

  ○ (2000) *Blood Press Suppl.* **2**: 21–4.

- HOPE (Heart Outcomes Prevention Study)

  ○ (2002) *NEJM.* **347**: 145–53.
  This study of ramipril showed a 32% decrease in stroke in patients with controlled BP, highlighting that all patients should have an ACE inhibitor irrespective of their BP.

- PROGRESS (Perindopril Protection Against Recurrent Strokes Study)

  ○ (2001) *Lancet.* **358**: 1033–41.
  One in 18 stroke sufferers who were treated with perindopril with or without indapamine avoided myocardial infarction, death or stroke over 5 years of treatment. The overall risk reduction was 26%.

Antiplatelet drugs
Aspirin is the treatment of choice for secondary prevention of stroke, especially for non-disabling stroke or transient ischaemic attack (13% reduction in subsequent events). No one dose is more effective than another (dispersible vs. enteric-coated efficacy is being debated).

- International Stroke Trial

  ○ (1997) *Lancet.* **349**: 1569–81.
  This trial used 300 mg aspirin.

- Antiplatelet Trialist Collaboration

  ○ (1994) *BMJ.* **308**: 81–106.
  Aspirin treatment that is started within 48 hours of an acute ischaemic stroke has been found to reduce the risk of both death and dependence, as does the continued use of aspirin. In high-risk patients (i.e. those with a history of prior ischaemic stroke), it reduced the odds of serious vascular events by 25%.

- Cochrane Review, 1999
  In this systemic review comparing thienopyridines (ticlopidone and clopidogrel) with aspirin, a further 12% absolute reduction in the odds of recurrent stroke was found.

- ESPS-2 (Second European Secondary Prevention Study)

○ (1999) *Arch Neurol.* **56**: 1087–92.
   Aspirin with dipyridamole 200 mg showed a small advantage over aspirin alone in decreasing stroke. There were wide confidence intervals (including no extra benefit). There was no effect on myocardial infarction or serious vascular events.

● ESPIRIT (European and Australian Stroke Prevention in Reversible Ischaemia Trial)
   The results of this trial are awaited.

● CAPRIE Study

○ (2002) Effectiveness of clopidogrel vs. aspirin in preventing acute MI in patients with symptomatic atherosclerosis. *Am J Cardiol.* **90**: 760–2.
   Clopidogrel inhibits platelet aggregation. In this secondary prevention study it showed a modest benefit over aspirin.

Anticoagulation in atrial fibrillation

Atrial fibrillation (AF) increases the risk of stroke sixfold.

Warfarin was previously the drug of choice for prevention of stroke. Several randomised controlled trials confirmed the benefit and low complication rate (0.4%). The number needed to treat was 11.

○ (2001) Systematic review of long-term anticoagulation of antiplatelet treatment in patients with non-rheumatic atrial fibrillation. *BMJ.* **322**: 321–6.
   This review found no added benefit in *non-rheumatic AF*. Previous meta-analyses had not included these trials. There were 3298 patients (thought to be too low a number, as around 5000 are needed). Individual trials were small and used slightly different international normalised ratios. Around 45% were more likely to bleed on warfarin (even within the controlled setting of the trial). It was concluded that there was no obvious benefit gained from using warfarin.

○ (2001) Comparison of warfarin and aspirin for the prevention of recurrent ischaemic strokes. *NEJM.* **345**: 1444–51.
   This study compared the use of aspirin with warfarin in non-cardiogenic causes of stroke. The two groups did not differ in overall rates of death or recurrent ischaemic stroke over a 2-year period.

Cholesterol

If a patient has had a stroke but does not have coronary heart disease (CHD), the benefits of a reduction in cholesterol levels are less clear. SPARCI and MRC/BHF are ongoing trials (not yet published) that should provide some answers.

○ (2002) *Lancet.* **360**: 7–20.

● The Heart Protection Study

○ (2002) *Lancet.* **360**: 7–20.
   This study of the treatment of high-risk CHD patients with simvastatin found that the latter reduced the incidence of stroke by up to 25%.

● Pravastatin therapy and risk of stroke

○ (2000) *NEJM.* **343**: 317–26.
   In this study, 9014 patients with myocardial infarction or unstable angina were randomised to pravastatin 40 mg or placebo. A reduced risk of stroke was found in the pravastatin group (relative risk reduction, 19%; $P = 0.05$). There was no effect on haemorrhagic stroke.

- CARE Study and 4S

These had similar findings, possibly due to progression of atherosclerosis, plaque stabilisation and improved endothelial function.

Specialised care

- Cochrane Review 1999
  A total of 19 randomised controlled trials involving 3864 patients were reviewed. After a 1-year follow-up, patients in stroke rehabilitation units had lower death rates and lower rates of dependency (30%) (i.e. patients were often living at home).

- Domiciliary occupational therapy

  ○ (2000) *BMJ.* **320**: 603–6.
    It was found that this service initially improved functional outcome and satisfaction after discharge. However, these benefits were not sustained.

The Royal College of Physicians published evidence-based national clinical guidelines for stroke management in 2000. The Action for Stroke Group (PO Box 31412, London W4 1FJ) has also published guidelines which are available from this address. They cover management issues, social aspects in terms of carers and families, occupational therapy, physiotherapy, speech therapy, etc. It is also important to look for evidence of cardiovascular disease, carotid artery stenosis, diabetes, smoking, obesity, etc., when managing the patient.

Carotid endarterectomy
If there is a symptomatic stenosis, the benefit of surgery relates to the degree of stenosis. This is classified as mild, moderate, or severe (Cochrane Review, 2003).
  Surgery is recommended within 6 months of the first symptoms appearing if there is a 70% stenosis (or more). It is not indicated for asymptomatic stenosis.
  Carotid Dopplers should be performed on all anterior circulation strokes.

Lifestyle changes
The most important of these is smoking cessation.

Miscellaneous

○ (2001) Effectiveness of home-based support for older people: systematic review. *BMJ.* **323**: 719–25.
  This study concluded that home visits to older people can reduce both mortality and the number of admissions to long-term institutional care.

○ (2002) The incidence of stroke and TIAs is falling: a report from the Belgian sentinel stations. *Br J Gen Pract.* **52**: 813–17.
  A Belgian network of GPs looked at four registration years between 1984 and 1999. A total of 1097 events were classified as stroke (total population covered was >500 000). In those over 60 years of age, a reduction of one-third in men and one-quarter in women was found. The reduction in transient ischaemic attacks was not significant. The improvement is thought to be due to improved prescribing in secondary prevention (e.g. aspirin, hypertension, encouraging lifestyle changes).

Diabetes

- The prevalence of diabetes in the UK is 3% (10% in those over 65 years of age).
- Life expectancy is reduced by up to 20 years in insulin-dependent diabetes mellitus (IDDM) and 10 years in non-insulin-dependent diabetes mellitus (NIDDM).
- Coronary heart disease is increased by fivefold and stroke is increased by threefold.

Diabetes is a complex multisystem disease, and for effective management you need, preferably, a co-ordinated patient-centred approach with set standards and a computerised register. It is a common disease, the incidence of which is rising due to the ageing population, obesity, sedentary lifestyle, etc. St Vincent's declaration, ratified by the WHO regional committee for Europe in 1991, set aspirations and goals for reducing the impact of diabetes.

Recent changes relating to diabetes include the following:

- new WHO classifications (June 2000)
- NICE guidelines
- the British Diabetic Association (BDA) has been renamed Diabetes UK
- the National Service Framework for diabetes.

Diagnosis

The criteria for diagnosis were agreed by the World Health Organization in June 2000.

1 Diabetic symptoms with random venous glucose concentration >11.1 mmol/L or fasting glucose BM > 7.0 mmol/L or 2-hour BM > 11.1 mmol/L after 75 g glucose tolerance test.

2 No symptoms – do not diagnose on the basis of a single glucose measurement, but do a repeat plasma test.

Patients should be classified according to pathological type (i.e. type 1 or 2) and then by stage (i.e. insulin dependent or not).

The implications of these changes are that more people will be diagnosed as being diabetic (most will be diet controlled). Hopefully, long-term complications will be reduced, but in the mean time the workload for primary care will be substantial.

Research presented at the European Association of Diabetes in September 2001 emphasised that even the new WHO guidelines on the oral glucose tolerance test (OGTT) (for those with plasma glucose levels in the range 6.1–6.9 mmol/L) would miss up to 20% of people with impaired glucose tolerance, and recommended that an OGTT should be performed at concentrations in the range 5.0–6.9 mmol/L. Even by using this range, 11% of diabetes cases would go undetected.

Obesity in diabetes

Up to 80% of type 2 diabetes is due to obesity (BMI > 27 kg/m^2); the duration of obesity is significant. Weight loss improves morbidity (UK Prospective Diabetes Study 7).

○ (2002) Reduction in the incidence of type 2 diabetes with lifestyle intervention or metformin. *NEJM.* **346**: 393–403.
This followed on from plans outlined by the Diabetes Prevention Programme in 1999. It was a RCT of 3234 non-diabetics and it found that lifestyle changes and treatment with metformin both reduced the incidence of diabetes. The lifestyle intervention was more effective than metformin.

○ (2001) Diet, lifestyle and the risk of type 2 diabetes mellitus in women. *NEJM.* **345**: 790–7.
A total of 84 941 female nurses aged 30–55 years were monitored from 1980 to 1996. An important risk factor was BMI > 35 kg/m^2. Poor diet, minimal exercise, smoking and abstinence from alcohol were all associated with a significant risk of developing diabetes. It comes as no great surprise that lifestyle is a key risk.

○ (2001) *Diabetic Care.* **25**: 148–98, 200–12.
This study gave revised recommendations on diet, emphasising total carbohydrate intake rather than control of high sugar content in food. It recommended that less than 10% of calories should be delivered from saturated fats, and that dietary cholesterol levels should be less than 300 mg/day.

○ (2001) Prevention of type 2 diabetes by changes in lifestyle among subjects with impaired glucose tolerance test. *NEJM.* **333**: 1343–50.
A randomised study of 522 middle-aged overweight people with an impaired glucose tolerance test showed that lifestyle changes can reduce the risk of progression of diabetes by 58% over 4 years.

HbA$_{1C}$ < 7.0: what is the evidence?

• Diabetes Control and Complications Trial (DCCT)

○ (2000) *NEJM.* **342**: 381–5 (the long-term follow-up publication).
A total of 1441 patients were followed over a period of 6.5 years while they received intensive treatment vs. conventional treatment. Intensive treatment improved microvascular and neuropathic complications, which correlates with decreased HbA$_{1C}$ levels. These patients did have more hypoglycaemic episodes (the results were less favourable in children under 13 years and adults over 70 years).

• UK Prospective Diabetes Study 33 (UKPDS 33)

○ (1998) *Lancet.* **352**: 837–53, 854–65.
The UKPDS is a large ongoing study of type 2 diabetes that has involved around 5000 patients since 1977. It looked at newly diagnosed diabetics and treated them with diet for three months. If their HbA$_{1C}$ level remained elevated, they were entered into the trial. It was found that intensive treatment (mean HbA$_{1C}$ 7% over the first 10 years) reduced the frequency of microvascular end points. In overweight patients with NIDDM, metformin and diet reduced the risk of diabetes-related end points by 32% and diabetic deaths by 42%. Blood pressure control ($<150/85$ mmHg) reduced microvascular complications and diabetes-related deaths (similar findings in the HOT Study: blood pressure $<130/80$ mmHg). Around 50% of diabetics had early signs of complications at the time of diagnosis (hence the importance of screening).

- UKPDS 63 and UKPDS 41

  o (2002) *BMJ*. **325**: 860–3.

  o (2000) *BMJ*. **320**: 1373–8.
    These studies concluded that the additional costs of intensive management are largely offset by a significant reduction in the costs of treating complications (estimated to be £695 per patient for treatment and £957 per patient for treatment of complications, hospital admissions, outpatient visits, eye and renal problems, etc.).

- UKPDS 35

  o (2000) *BMJ*. **321**: 405–12.
    Each 1% reduction in HbA_{1C} was associated with risk a reduction of 21% for diabetic end points; 21% related to diabetic deaths, 14% to myocardial infarction and 37% to microvascular complications.

  o (2001) The case against aggressive treatment of type 2 diabetes: critique of UKPDS. *BMJ*. **323**: 854–8.
    The UKPDS grew out of the authors' interest in the use of basal rather than postprandial glucose. The first report was published in 1983. During the course of the study, the length of the follow-up has changed, the end points have been redefined, the study is no longer blinded, the statistical analyses used have been questioned, and the changes have not been consistent with scientific principles.

Hypertension in diabetes

Around 70% of adults with NIDDM have hypertension and more than 70% have raised cholesterol levels.

- UKPDS 36 (and 49)

  o (2000) *BMJ*. **321**: 412–19.
    'In type 2 diabetes, the risk of diabetic complications is strongly associated with raised BP. Any reduction in BP is likely to reduce the risk of complications. The lowest risk seen is in those diabetics with a systolic BP < 120 mmHg.'
    Intensive blood pressure control is at least as important (if not more so) than intensive blood glucose level control.

British Hypertension Society guidelines based on the Hypertension Optimal Treatment Randomised Trial, 2000

- Start treatment at >140 mmHg systolic blood pressure and >90 mmHg diastolic blood pressure.

- Aim for a value of 130/80 mmHg, or 125/75 mmHg if there is proteinuria.

- Less than 30% of cases respond to monotherapy.

- *Do not forget* non-pharmacological treatment.

It is estimated that the number of diabetics on anti-hypertensives would need to double in order to meet targets of 140/80 mmHg.

- UKPDS 36

  o (2000) *BMJ*. **321**: 412–19.
  For systolic blood pressure, each 10 mmHg decrease is associated with a risk reduction of 12% for any complications related to diabetes (15% for deaths related to diabetes, 11% for myocardial infarction and 13% for microvascular complications).

Trials

- ### Hypertension Optimal Treatment (HOT) Randomised Trial

  o (1998) Effects of intensive blood pressure lowering and low-dose aspirin in patients with hypertension: principle results of the Hypertension Optimal Treatment Randomised Trial. *Lancet*. **351**: 1755–62. The results showed low rates of cardiovascular events if raised blood pressure was lowered. There were benefits of lowering diastolic blood pressure to 82.6 mmHg, and there was a 50% decrease in major cardiovascular events with a target diastolic blood pressure of 80 mmHg in diabetics compared with 90 mmHg.
  Acetylsalicylic acid reduced major cardiovascular events, especially myocardial infarction. There was no effect on the incidence of stroke or fatal bleeding, and non-fatal major bleeds were twice as common.

- ### HOPE and Micro-HOPE (Health Outcome Prevention Evaluation)

  o (2000) Effects of ramipril on cardiovascular and microvascular outcomes in people with diabetes mellitus. *Lancet*. **355**: 253–9.
  A total of 3577 diabetics aged 55 years or over were randomised to ramipril 10 mg/day or placebo and vitamin E or placebo. Ramipril had a beneficial effect on cardiovascular events, which decreased by 25–30%, and on overt nephropathy in people with diabetes. The benefit was greater than that attributable to the decrease in blood pressure. Vasculoprotective and renoprotective effects of ramipril in diabetics were seen.

- ### CALM (Candesartan and Lisinopril Microalbuminuria) study

  o (2000) Randomised controlled trial of dual blockade of renin–angiotensin system in patients with hypertension, microalbuminuria and NIDDM. The Candesartan and Lisinopril Microalbuminuria study. *BMJ*. **321**: 1440–4.
  In this prospective randomised double-blind study of 199 patients aged 30–75 years, candesartan 16 mg OD was as effective as lisinopril 20 mg OD in reducing blood pressure and microalbuminuria in hypertensive patients with type II diabetes. Combination treatment was well tolerated and was more effective in reducing blood pressure.

- ### EUCLID (Eurodiab Controlled Trial of Lisinopril in IDDM) trial

  o (1997) *Lancet*. **349**: 1787–92.
  In this multinational multicentre randomised double-blind placebo-controlled parallel-group trial, lisinopril slowed the progression of renal disease in normotensive IDDM patients with little or no albuminuria, although the greatest effect was in those with microalbuminuria ($>20\ \mu g$/min).

- ### BRILLIANT (Blood Pressure, Renal effects, Insulin control, Lipids, Lisinopril and Nifedipine Trial)

  o (1996) *J Hum Hypertens*. **10**: 185–92.
  In this multicentre randomised double-blind parallel-group trial, lisinopril was more effective than nifedipine in decreasing urinary albumin excretion.

- SYST-EUR (SHEP Co-operative Research Group)

  o (1988) *J Clin Epidemiol.* **41**: 197–208.
    With nitrendipine and enalapril vs. thiazide, the excess risk of diabetes was almost completely elimi-nated as a result of antihypertensive treatment.

  o (2002) Effects of losartan on renal and cardiovascular outcomes in patients with type 2 diabetes and nephropathy. *NEJM.* **345**: 861–9.
    Losartan was found to reduce the risk of end-stage renal disease by 28%, a level beyond that attribu-table to blood pressure control, in patients with type 2 diabetes and nephropathy.

  o RENAAL, IDNT, IRMA 2

  o (2002) The role of angiotensin II antagonism in type 2 diabetes: a review of renoprotective studies. *Clin Ther.* **24**(7): 1019–34.
    This review looked at:
    – RENAAL (reduction in end points in NIDDM with angiotensin II antagonist losartan). Found losartan to be renoprotective beyond that found with BP control.
    – IDNT (ibesartan diabetic nephropathy trial).
    – IRMA 2 (ibesartan in patients with type 2 diabetes and microalbuminuria study). Both found similar effects with ibesartan as had been found with losartan.

National Service Framework for Diabetes (2003 Delivery Strategy)

www.doh.gov.uk/nsf/diabetes/

This document states that 'all adults with diabetes will receive high-quality care throughout their lifetime, including support to optimise the control of their blood sugar'.
   It includes 12 standards in nine areas of diabetic care.

1 *Prevention of type 2 diabetes*
  - Multi-agency approach to reduce the number of people who are inactive, overweight and obese.
  - Physical education and a balanced diet need to be promoted from childhood.

2 *Identification of people with diabetes*
  Follow-up of those at increased risk (gestational diabetics, known family history, ischaemic heart disease, obesity and ethnicity).

3 *Empowering people with diabetes*
  - Has been shown to reduce blood glucose levels and improve quality of life.
  - Could involve structured education, personal care plans and patient-held records.

4 *Clinical care of adults with diabetes*
  Would include management of diabetes, hypertension and smoking cessation, all aimed at improving measurements and quality of life.

5 and 6 *Clinical care of children and young people with diabetes*
  Similar high-quality care to that for adults. It would also include physical, psychological, intellectual, educational and social development needs.

7 *Management of diabetic emergencies*
Diabetic ketoacidosis (DKA), hyperosmolar non-ketotic syndrome (HONK) and hypoglycaemia.

8 *Care of people with diabetes during admission to hospital*
Outcome could be improved by better communication between the diabetes team and ward staff.

9 *Diabetes and pregnancy*
Policies will be developed for women with pre-existing diabetes and those who develop diabetes, to help to achieve blood pressure control before and during pregnancy.

10, 11 and 12 *Detection and management of long-term complications*
 • Regular surveillance for long-term complications.
 • Effective treatment and investigation of complications.
 • Integrated health and social care.

Delivery strategy

1 Primary care trusts will set local priorities.

2 The NSF standards will be rolled out in conjunction with NICE guidelines.

3 By 2006, a minimum of 80% of diabetics should be offered screening for early detection of retinopathy (digital retinal photography). This figure should rise to 100% by 2007. Standards will be set by the National Screening Committee.

4 Primary care priorities are as follows:
 • updating of practice registers
 • patients to be given appropriate advice on diet, physical activity, smoking and treatment in line with the National Service Framework.

5 The personal diabetes record and agreed care plan includes the following:
 • education and personal goals of the person with diabetes
 • how the diabetes will be managed until the next review, and a named contact.

○ (2001) Randomised controlled trial of structured personal care of type 2 diabetes. *BMJ.* **323**: 970–5.
 This trial showed that structured personal care programmes lower risk factors for complications in people with type 2 diabetes. The programmes involved regular follow-up, individual goal setting supported by prompting by doctors, clinical guidelines, feedback and continuing medical education.

○ (2002) Effective diabetes care: a need for realistic targets. *BMJ.* **324**: 1577–80.
 Aggressive treatment of hyperglycaemia, dyslipidaemia and hypertension as well as the regular use of antiplatelet agents has been advocated in type 2 diabetes. Current targets are attainable in only 50–70% of individuals. Targets are often impractical and involve so many drugs that the patient will not comply with treatment. Individually tailored targets are needed, and their effectiveness will be shown by an improvement in diabetes clinics.

○ (2001) Management of diabetes: are doctors framing the benefits from the wrong perspective? *BMJ.* **323**: 994–6.

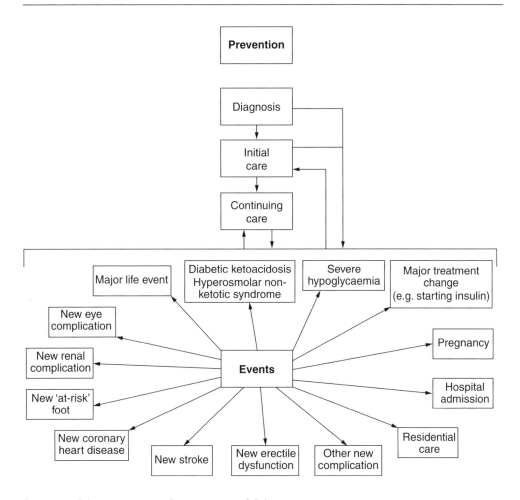

Summary of the prevention and management of diabetes

In the old treatment framework, tight glycaemic control is the primary end point, and the focus is on organising life routines and eating patterns around insulin-injection profiles. The implicit message is that good diabetes control is synonymous with giving up flexibility and choice – that is, allowing diabetes to control your life.

o (2002) Training in flexible intensive insulin management to enable dietary freedom in people with type 1 diabetes: Dose Adjustments For Normal Eating (DAFNE) randomised controlled trial. *BMJ.* **325**: 746–9.

This secondary care study in the UK looked at 169 adults with type 1 diabetes with moderate or poor glycaemic control. It was found that at 6 months the group that had been given training that promoted dietary freedom had a better quality of life and better glycaemic control (mean HbA$_{1C}$ of 8.4% compared with 9.4% in the non-trained group), and the number of hypoglycaemic episodes was no higher.

The DAFNE programme offers a 1-week intensive training course in small groups working with specialist nurses and dietitians. The course would cost £500 and is awaiting consideration by NICE.

The new treatment framework for diabetes can be summarised as follows.

1 Tools of intensive management are presented as a means to increase freedom in a patient's life.

2 The focus is on developing an insulin regimen that is flexible and fits in with the demands of life.

3 The implicit message is that you can achieve good diabetes control without having to yield control of your life to diabetes.

NICE guidelines on the management of type 2 diabetes

Management of blood glucose levels

- HbA_{1C} should be measured 2 to 6-monthly and should be in the range 6.5–7.5%.

- Weight loss and physical activity should be encouraged if the patient is overweight.

Management of blood pressure and lipids

- An annual risk assessment should be made if there is no ischaemic heart disease.

- Blood pressure should be checked yearly; if $>140/80$ mmHg or $<160/100$ mmHg, recommend lifestyle changes, repeat after 6 months. If it is $>140/80$ mmHg and there is a high 10-year coronary risk or albuminuria, start treatment.

- Measure lipids yearly; if raised cholesterol >5 mmol/L and triglyceride >2.3 mmol/L ask for advice and treat if there is an inadequate response.

Glitazones/thiazolidinediones

Since the withdrawal of Troglitazone (within 6 weeks of its launch in 1997) because it had been found to cause severe liver damage in a few patients, two new drugs have recently been licensed in the UK for treatment of type 2 diabetes, namely rosiglitazone (Avandia) and pioglitazone (Actos). These drugs enhance the effects of insulin in adipose tissue and skeletal muscle.

○ (2001) *Drug Ther Bull.* **39**: 65–7.
   This article gives a sensible overview.

The NICE guidelines (August 2003) state that these drugs are for use with metformin (especially in cases of obesity) or sulphonylureas. They are not licensed in the UK for triple therapy, monotherapy or use with insulin. An increased incidence of cardiac failure has been observed with rosiglitazone when used with insulin. Pioglitazone has been licensed for use with insulin in the USA. Both drugs have been approved for monotherapy.

○ (2000) *BMJ.* **321**: 252–3.

Although they appear to be safe, it is recommended that liver function tests are performed prior to starting treatment and then at two-monthly intervals for the first year, stopping the drug if the liver enzymes rise to three times their normal level or if the patient becomes jaundiced.

The *Drug and Therapeutics Bulletin* has attacked NICE recommendations on the grounds that they go beyond what is in the licence (which states that they should only be given to the obese and those who cannot take metformin). NICE has responded by saying that the *Drug and Therapeutics Bulletin* is not privy to the same information and that they only look at things from a clinical perspective, whereas NICE considers all angles.

Meglitinides/prandial glucose regulators

These include nateglinide, rateglinide and repaglinide. They are amino-acid derivatives which are licensed for use with metformin in patients with type 2 diabetes, where better control is needed (i.e. $HbA_{1C} > 7.5\%$), or in cases where patients experience hypoglycaemia when treated with sulphonylureas. Repaglinide is licensed for monotherapy.

The drugs are 'glucose responsive', so they induce insulin release when the patient eats by acting on the pancreatic beta-cells to stimulate a rapid, short-lived release of insulin to a level that is dependent on the glucose concentration (i.e. where there is a postprandial rise in glucose level). This is beneficial if the patient has an erratic lifestyle (e.g. junior doctors). As stimulation is not over 24 hours, the endocrine function should be preserved.

○ DECODE Study Group (1999) Glucose tolerance and mortality: comparison of WHO and American Diabetes Association diagnostic criteria. *Lancet*. **354**: 617–21.
This study of 18 048 men and 7316 women aged over 30 years looked at the risk of death according to different diagnostic glucose categories, with a follow-up period of 7.3 years. It found that fasting glucose alone did not identify the risk of death associated with hyperglycaemia. Mortality increased with increasing 2-hour glucose (i.e. postprandial spike).

Screening

Mass population screening would be costly and inefficient with a low specificity, as less than 1% of undiagnosed cases were revealed by a British Diabetic Association study in 1994. Many organisations have published arguments for a targeted approach to high-risk groups (e.g. the obese, family history of diabetes, ethnic groups, and patients with gestational diabetes, impaired glucose tolerance or hypertension).

○ (2001) Should we screen for type 2 diabetes? Evaluation against National Screening Committee Criteria. *BMJ*. **322**: 986–8.
This discussion paper looks at the role of the National Screening Committee in evaluating a screening programme for type 2 diabetes. It summarises as follows.

• The benefits of early detection and treatment of undiagnosed diabetes have not been proved.

- The disadvantages of screening are important and should be quantified.

- Universal screening is not merited, but targeted screening may be justified.

- Clinical management of diabetes should be optimised before a screening programme is considered.
  No agreement was reached on how targeted screening could be achieved. A further report is expected in 2005.

  o (2001) Screening for diabetes in general practice: cross-sectional population study. *BMJ.* **323**: 548–51.
    This study concluded that although it is feasible to use age as a sole risk factor, this has a low yield, and it recommends screening targeted at patients with multiple risk factors.

Diabetes UK (formerly the British Diabetic Association) recommends opportunistic screening for those at high risk of diabetes.

  o (2002) Targeting people with pre-diabetes (editorial). *BMJ.* **325**: 403–40.
    This considers lifestyle changes and the evidence that supports investment in these changes.

Miscellaneous

Acarbose

  o (2002) Acarbose for prevention of type 2 diabetes mellitus: the STOP-NIDDM randomised trial. *Lancet.* **359**: 2072–7.
    People with impaired glucose tolerance who were treated with acarbose were 25% less likely to develop type 2 diabetes than those on placebo. It was concluded that acarbose could be used either as an alternative or in addition to lifestyle changes in patients with impaired glucose tolerance.

Vitamin D

  o (2001) *Lancet.* **358**: 1500–3.
    In this longitudinal study of 10 366 children which was conducted between 1966 and 1997, children who were given vitamin D (irrespective of dose) had a lower rate of type 2 diabetes. This suggests that it is important to ensure infants get at least the recommended daily allowance of vitamin D.

Vaccine

  o (2001) *Lancet.* **358**: 1749–53.
    DiaPep277 is the first drug to successfully halt the immune system's destruction of pancreatic beta-cells. However, the intervals at which the vaccine should be given are not yet known. Phase III trials are about to begin.

Respiratory disorders

Asthma

- Around 5.4% of the population are estimated to have asthma (by the National Asthma Campaign).

- The proportion diagnosed in children rose from 4% to 10% between 1964 and 1989.

- Around 1500 deaths per year are due to acute asthma.

- The annual cost of asthma to the NHS is £700 million (this does not include the economic cost of working days lost).

- Children who were exposed to antibiotics *in utero* are thought to be more likely to develop asthma (by up to 43%), hayfever (up to 38%) and eczema (up to 11%). However, this has only been shown in one study.

Although the British Thoracic Society guidelines have been successful, asthma is still under-diagnosed and under-treated.

A recent Government inquiry into asthma deaths concluded that many of them could have been prevented by more proactive GP care. It cited the following problems:

- under-use of primary care services

- under-prescribing of oral steroids

- inadequate use of peak expiratory flow rate (PEFR).

It also found that only 12% of those who had died had attended a practice asthma clinic during the year before their death.

○ (2000) Validity of symptom and clinical measures of asthma severity for primary outpatient assessment of adult asthma. *Br J Gen Pract.* **50**: 7–12.
This study looked at symptom-based assessment of asthma and found it to be useful, but obviously still advocated the use of PEFR. Questions that were used included the following. Have you had difficulty sleeping because of your asthma? Have you experienced your asthma symptoms during the day? Has your asthma interfered with your usual activities?

○ (2003) Accessibility, acceptability and effectiveness in primary care of routine telephone review of asthma: pragmatic randomised controlled trial. *BMJ.* **326**: 4776–9.
In this randomised trial involving 278 patients, most people who were reviewed by telephone showed no clinical disadvantage or loss of satisfaction.

○ (1999) Guided self-management of asthma: how to do it. *BMJ.* **319**: 759–60.
This clinical review reached the following conclusions:
  – Self-management prevents exacerbations, improves care and is cost-effective.
  – Patient education is crucial, and should be given in a structured way.
  – Patients should be taught to understand their symptoms and monitor their PEFR at home.
  – Patients should know how to act when signs of asthma deterioration first appear.
  – There should always be supervision and continuity in asthma care.

There is plenty of evidence that self-management reduces hospital admission rates and time off work, and improves symptoms.

- ○ (2000) *BMJ*. **321**: 1507–10.
  Interestingly, this article showed that many patients believed they were already managing their asthma and were not otherwise interested. They did not regard asthma as a chronic disease, and preferred to manage it acutely.

Leukotriene-receptor antagonists

These are derived from arachidonic acid, the precursor of prostaglandins. By preventing prostaglandin release, they reduce bronchoconstriction, mucus secretion and oedema.

- COMPACT Trial

- ○ (2003) *Thorax*. **58**: 211–16.
  This multinational trial compared the addition of montelukast 10 mg/day to doubling the steroid dose in 889 adults with asthma. Lung function improved earlier with montelukast, but after 6 weeks both stategies had worked.

- ○ (1999) Randomised controlled trial of effect of a leukotriene-receptor agonist, montelukast, on tapering inhaled corticosteroids in asthmatic patients. *BMJ*. **319**: 87–90.
  This trial showed that montelukast reduced the need for inhaled corticosteroids to maintain asthma control.

Leukotriene-receptor antagonists are licensed as add-on therapy in moderate to severe asthmatics (i.e. steps 3 to 4 in the BTS guidelines).

Chlorofluorocarbon (CFC)-free inhalers

- CFCs have implications for the depletion of the ozone layer.

- They can be used as propellants in metered-dose inhalers.

- CFC-free metered-dose inhalers have been available since 1995 in the UK, and are now being widely used.

- Hydrofluoroalkane (HFA) compounds are being used in preference; their safety profile is similar to that of CFCs.

- The change to CFC-free inhalers is taking longer than anticipated because of drug formulations and practical problems.

Long-acting beta-2 agonists

- MIASMA (Meta-analysis of increased dose of inhaled steroid or addition of salmeterol in symptomatic asthma)

○ (2000) *BMJ.* **320**: 1368–73.
   Lung function was higher in patients who received salmeterol rather than steroids. Symptom-free days and nights were more frequent with salmeterol, as were rescue-free days and nights. There was less exacerbation of symptoms with salmeterol, and the severity was less in those who did experience this.

Breathing exercises

As yet there is no reliable body of evidence to indicate whether breathing exercises work for asthma (Cochrane Review, 2001), although it would make sense if they did.

Scottish Intercollegiate Guidelines Network/BTS Asthma Guidelines

○ (2003) *Thorax.* **58** (Suppl. 1).
   www.brit-thoracic.org.uk

These guidelines have now been updated from the 1995 guidelines. Their aims are to achieve accurate diagnosis and control symptoms quickly by stepping up treatment, and subsequently stepping down treatment when control is good.

   The guidelines are broken down into those for adults, children aged 5–12 years and children under 5 years. They suggest that there should be a method for identification of poorly controlled asthmatics so that they can be asked to come in, or chased up if they do not attend, as there is a higher mortality rate in this group.

Step 1: short-acting bronchodilators (beta-2 agonists, ipratropium)

Step 2: introduction of a regular preventor (dose appropriate for disease severity)
There is no additional benefit in starting high and stepping down.
   Inhaled steroids are the first choice. Alternatives include the following:

• cromones (sodium cromoglycate)

• leukotriene-receptor antagonists

• theophyllines

• long-acting beta-2 agonists.

Step 3: add-on therapy
Long acting beta-2 agonists are used. If the response remains suboptimal, increase the inhaled steroid dose to:

• 800 μg/day in adults

• 400 μg/day in children aged 5–12 years.

Consider further add-ons (cf. Step 2).

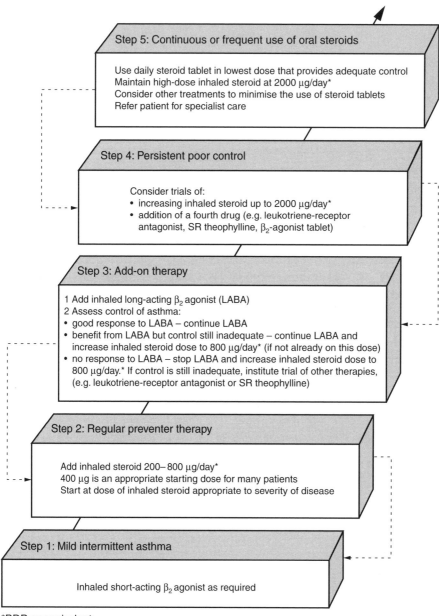

Step 5: Continuous or frequent use of oral steroids

Use daily steroid tablet in lowest dose that provides adequate control
Maintain high-dose inhaled steroid at 2000 µg/day*
Consider other treatments to minimise the use of steroid tablets
Refer patient for specialist care

Step 4: Persistent poor control

Consider trials of:
• increasing inhaled steroid up to 2000 µg/day*
• addition of a fourth drug (e.g. leukotriene-receptor
  antagonist, SR theophylline, β_2-agonist tablet)

Step 3: Add-on therapy

1 Add inhaled long-acting β_2 agonist (LABA)
2 Assess control of asthma:
• good response to LABA – continue LABA
• benefit from LABA but control still inadequate – continue LABA and
  increase inhaled steroid dose to 800 µg/day* (if not already on this dose)
• no response to LABA – stop LABA and increase inhaled steroid dose to
  800 µg/day.* If control is still inadequate, institute trial of other therapies,
  (e.g. leukotriene-receptor antagonist or SR theophylline)

Step 2: Regular preventer therapy

Add inhaled steroid 200– 800 µg/day*
400 µg is an appropriate starting dose for many patients
Start at dose of inhaled steroid appropriate to severity of disease

Step 1: Mild intermittent asthma

Inhaled short-acting β_2 agonist as required

*BDP or equivalent.

Summary of the stepwise management of asthma in adults

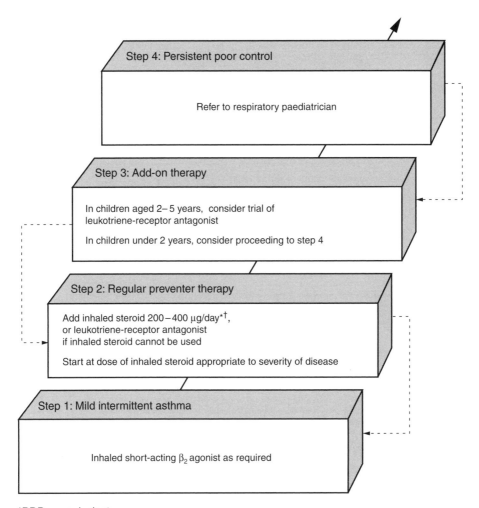

*BDP or equivalent.
†Higher nominal doses may be required if drug delivery is difficult.

Summary of the stepwise management of asthma in children under 5 years of age

Step 4: addition of a fourth drug

If there is poor control of symptoms on a moderate dose of inhaled steroid and add-on therapy, consider the following:

• increasing steroids to 2000 µg/day in adults or 800 µg/day in children aged 5–12 years

• leukotriene-receptor antagonists

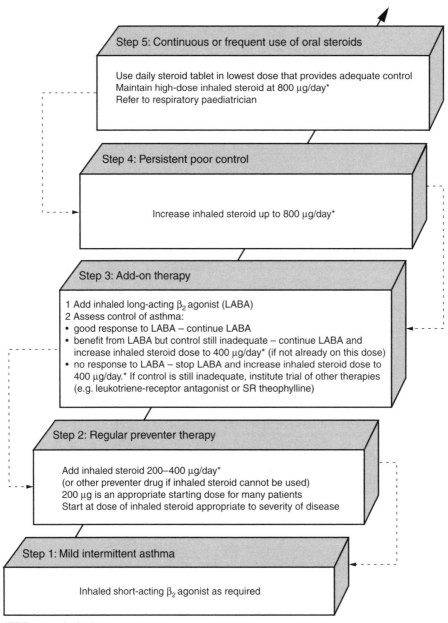

Step 5: Continuous or frequent use of oral steroids

Use daily steroid tablet in lowest dose that provides adequate control
Maintain high-dose inhaled steroid at 800 µg/day*
Refer to respiratory paediatrician

Step 4: Persistent poor control

Increase inhaled steroid up to 800 µg/day*

Step 3: Add-on therapy

1 Add inhaled long-acting β_2 agonist (LABA)
2 Assess control of asthma:
• good response to LABA – continue LABA
• benefit from LABA but control still inadequate – continue LABA and
  increase inhaled steroid dose to 400 µg/day* (if not already on this dose)
• no response to LABA – stop LABA and increase inhaled steroid dose to
  400 µg/day.* If control is still inadequate, institute trial of other therapies
  (e.g. leukotriene-receptor antagonist or SR theophylline)

Step 2: Regular preventer therapy

Add inhaled steroid 200–400 µg/day*
(or other preventer drug if inhaled steroid cannot be used)
200 µg is an appropriate starting dose for many patients
Start at dose of inhaled steroid appropriate to severity of disease

Step 1: Mild intermittent asthma

Inhaled short-acting β_2 agonist as required

*BDP or equivalent.

Summary of the stepwise management of asthma in children aged 5 to 12 years

- theophyllines
- slow-release beta-2 agonist tablets.

If an addition is ineffective, stop it or reduce it back to the original dose.

Step 5: continuous or frequent use of oral steroids
This is defined as more than 3 months' continuous treatment or three to four courses per year.

- Immunosuppressants (methotrexate, cyclosporin and oral gold), 3-month trial.
- Continuous subcutaneous terbutaline infusion.

Organisation of care
All practices should have a list of patients with asthma.

Review
- This should be routine with a standard recording system.
- It should include inhaler technique, PEFR, current treatment, morbidity and asthma action plan.
- It should be audited regularly.
- The best results are seen with nurses who have been trained in asthma management.

The following three questions should be asked:

1 Do you have you difficulty sleeping because of your asthma?
2 Have you experienced your asthma symptoms during the day?
3 Has your asthma interfered with your usual activities?

Asthma action plans
- These should be customised and written.
- They should be offered to all patients with asthma.

Acute exacerbations
- Inpatients should be on specialist units.
- Discharge should be a planned and supervised event. It may take place as soon as clinical improvement is apparent.

Targeting care
Identify groups at risk. They include the following:

- children with frequent upper respiratory tract infections
- children over 5 years of age with persistent symptoms
- asthmatics with psychiatric disorders or learning disability
- patients who are using large quantities of beta-2 agonists.

Main changes from 1995 guidelines

- Asthma action plans are advocated.
- Long-acting bronchodilators are now recommended as the preferred additional therapy before increasing inhaled steroids. Leukotriene-receptor antagonists are also advocated.
- Inhaled steroids are tailored to the disease; there is no advantage starting with a high dose and stepping down.

Chronic obstructive pulmonary/airways disease

British Thoracic Society (BTS) definition

'A chronic slowly progressive disorder characterised by airflow obstruction that does not change markedly over several months. Most of the lung function is fixed, although some reversibility can be produced by bronchodilator (or other) therapy.'

- Chronic obstructive pulmonary disease (COPD) causes around 26 000 deaths per year (respiratory disease is now the biggest killer in the UK).
- It is responsible for 400–1000 per 10 000 consultations in general practice.
- Risk factors include smoking, pollution, occupation (cadmium and coal related), lower social classes, genetic factors, and chronic under-treatment of asthma.

The BTS published guidelines in 1997 aimed at improving diagnosis and management.

○ (1997) *Thorax*. **52** (Suppl. 5): S1–28.

GOLD have also published COPD guidelines at www.goldcopd.com.

Diagnosis

This is suggested by symptoms and established by objective measurements using spirometry, with a chest X-ray to exclude other pathologies.

Spirometry is the only successful means of confirming a diagnosis and assessing severity. In October 2001, *GP News* looked at the potential savings that could be made by identifying COPD patients on asthma registers and withdrawing inhaled steroids (following data presented at the Eleventh European Respiratory Society Conference).

○ (1999) An observational study of inhaled corticosteroid withdrawal in stable COPD. *Resp Med*. **93**: 161–6.
This study pointed out the risk of exacerbation when stopping inhaled corticosteroids, and advocated careful monitoring.

A trial of steroids (30 mg prednisolone for 2 weeks, or 6 weeks of beclomethasone 1000 µg per day) is recommended when looking for reversibility. Reversibility is an increase of FEV_1 by 15% and 200 ml above the baseline.

Steroid use in COPD

- ISOLDE (Inhaled Steroids in Obstructive Lung Disease)

○ (2000) *BMJ*. **320**: 1297–303.
This randomised double-blind placebo-controlled trial looked at fluticasone 500 µg twice a day vs. placebo. Patients on fluticasone had a higher FEV_1, but the rate of lung function decline was the same in both groups. Patients on fluticasone had fewer exacerbations and showed a slower decline in overall health status.

- TRISTAN (Trial of Inhaled Steroids and Long-Acting Beta-2 Agonists)

○ (2003) *Lancet*. **361**: 449–56.
In this trial of 1465 patients, after 12 months of combined treatment (salmeterol and fluticasone) there was a significantly greater improvement in lung function than with either monotherapy or placebo. Combined treatment was also associated with the greatest reduction in symptoms.

○ (2003) *Eur Resp J*. **21**: 1–7.
This study found that a medium to high dose of inhaled steroids lowered the risk of mortality.

There is growing evidence that oral steroids help exacerbations (Cochrane Review, 2001). One randomised controlled trial showed that a 10-day course was better than 3 days of treatment. One review suggested that oral steroids decreased the length of hospital stay by 1–2 days, and this was not at the expense of raised blood sugar levels or secondary infections.

Smoking cessation (see overleaf)

This reduces the rate of decline in lung function.

○ Peto *et al*. (1977) *BMJ*. **1**: 1645–8.

Long-term oxygen therapy

In hypoxaemic patients, this prolongs life.

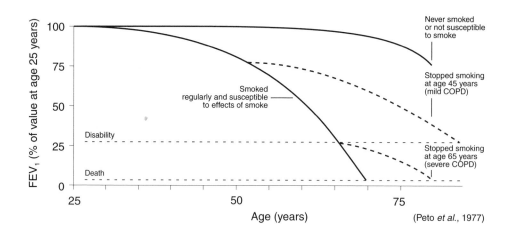

(Peto *et al.*, 1977)

- MRC trial

o (1981) *Lancet.* i: 681–6.
  This trial showed that five patients would need to be treated for 5 years in order to avoid one death (i.e. NNT = 5), where treatment involved administration of oxygen for 15 hours per day. The difference was only evident after 500 hours.

o (1980) *Ann Intern Med.* **93**: 391–8.
  In a trial of continuous vs. nocturnal oxygen, it was found that the risk of death was slightly higher if patients were receiving only nocturnal oxygen.

Both of the above trials form part of the evidence base for the BTS guidelines. Consider patients with cyanosis and cor pulmonale for long-term oxygen therapy assessment. This treatment should be considered if $PaO_2 < 7.3$ kPa, but it is important to ensure that it does not cause carbon dioxide retention. It should be prescribed for 15–20 hours per day.

It is worth noting that the 'as needed' use of oxygen cylinders represents one of the largest costs of COPD to the NHS. Although it provides symptomatic relief, there is no evidence to support its use. (Does this matter if the patient experiences symptom relief?)

N-acetylcysteine

This is a mucolytic agent that has been found to reduce the exacerbations of COPD (NNT = 6). It may also slow the rate of decline in lung function. It is now licensed in the UK.

Miscellaneous

o (2002) Randomised controlled trial of home-based care of patients with COPD. *BMJ.* **325**: 938–40.
  This trial found that brief intervention by community nurses after acute care improved knowledge and some aspects of quality of life, but failed to prevent presentation and readmission to hospital.

○ (2000) Hospital at home vs. hospital care in COPD: randomised controlled trial. *BMJ.* **321**: 1265–8.
  This trial randomised patients who would have been admitted after medical assessment in Accident and Emergency to either admission or nurse-administered home care. It is the first trial to show that hospital-at-home care can be as effective as inpatient care in some exacerbations.

Pulmonary rehabilitation

This can reduce symptoms, increase mobility and improve quality of life.

○ (2001) *Drug Ther Bull.* **39**: 81–4.

Exercise can reduce the risk of relapses that require hospital admission by 50%.

○ (2003) *Thorax.* **58**: 100–5.

Long-acting anticholinergics: tiotropium (launched in the UK in October 2002)

A once-daily maintenance dose for COPD has been shown to improve FEV_1 compared with placebo, salmeterol and ipratropium.

Osteoporosis

There is a higher risk of osteoporosis in COPD (compared with asthma), even when patients have not received long-term steroid treatment.

○ (2003) *Chest.* **122**: 1949–55.

Influenza

It is estimated that flu causes 2000–4000 deaths per year, mainly during a 6 to 8-week period over the winter.

○ (1991) *Br J Gen Pract.* **49**: 281–4.
  It has been shown that patients worry about getting a cold from the vaccine, but they do not believe that they are at risk of dying of flu.

Immunisation

Immunisation of those at high risk of serious illness from influenza reduces hospital admissions and deaths.

○ (1997) *Epidemiol Infect.* **118**: 27–33

○ (1995) *Epidemiol Infect.* **346**: 591–5.
  Immunisation can reduce mortality by up to 40%, and even up to 70% in repeated vaccination. It can reduce respiratory illness by up to 50%.

In the *CMO Update* May 2000, the vaccination programme was widened to include the following:

• all members of the population over 65 years of age

- all high-risk groups (cardiovascular disease, diabetes, immune suppression and chronic disease)

- all those in long-stay residential and nursing homes, as well as other long-stay facilities.

The health authorities were set targets of 70%, flu co-ordinators were appointed, and a major public health campaign was undertaken. Overall a 65% response rate was achieved in those over 65 years of age.

CMO immunisation programme 2001/2002

- A minimum target of 65% in those over 65 years of age was set.

- There was no change in the target groups.

- NHS employers should offer the vaccination to employees directly involved in patient care through the occupational health service, not their own GPs (unless they had been specifically contracted).

Patients who decline flu vaccination:

- consider influenza to be a mild disease (as it causes 3000–4000 deaths per year in the UK, it is more of an epidemic)

- hope they won't get flu

- doubt the effectiveness of the vaccine

- fear the side-effects of the vaccine, and think that it will give them flu (in fact, all vaccines can cause a flu-like illness as a side-effect)

- lack campaign awareness

- are apathetic

- are unable to attend (e.g. because they are housebound or in residential care)

- find the timing of immunisation clinics inconvenient

- lack information about the vaccination.

○ (2002) Boosting influenza immunisation for >65. *Br J Gen Pract.* **52**: 710–11.

○ (2000) *Br J Gen Pract.* **50**: 27–30.
   This study confirmed the safety of the vaccine in asthmatics, and highlighted the poor uptake in this important subgroup.

○ (1997) *Br J Gen Pract.* **47**: 363–6.
   A study from The Netherlands showed improved uptake in high-risk patients using personal reminders, computer-based records and monitoring of patient compliance.

○ (2002) Boosting uptake of influenza immunisation: a randomised controlled trial of telephone appointments in general practice. *Br J Gen Pract.* **52**: 712–16.
   This study showed that inner-city uptake was improved by 6% when receptionists arranged appointments by telephone. This was in a low-risk older population and has cost implications.

○ (2002) Improving uptake of influenza vaccination among older people: a randomised controlled trial. *Br J Gen Pract.* **52**: 717–21.
This study found that combining home-based over-75 checks with influenza vaccination can improve uptake.

Pneumococcal vaccine

This is a one-off vaccination (revaccinate after 5–10 years if antibody levels are likely to have declined). It can be given at the same time as the influenza vaccination, but at different sites.

Zanamivir (Relenza)

This neuraminidase inhibitor inhibits the replication of influenza A and B. It should be started within 48 hours of symptoms appearing, and is designed to complement the vaccination programme. Amantadine has been available since the 1970s, but is only effective against influenza A. Glaxo-Wellcome have conducted a number of trials, only a few of which have been published.

○ (1997) *NEJM.* **337**: 874–80.
In a study of 262 patients (in Europe and the USA), Relenza reduced the number of days of illness from 7 to 4 if taken within 30 hours. High-risk populations were not studied.

● MIST Study Group
In a study of 455 patients over 12 years of age, 76 individuals were high risk. Relenza reduced the length of the illness to an average of 2 days if taken within 36 hours.

○ (1998) Randomised trial of efficacy and safety of inhaled zanamivir. The MIST (Management of Influenza in the Southern Hemisphere Trialists) Study Group. *Lancet.* **352**: 1877–81.

● Health Technology Assessment Report (December 2000)
This meta-analysis of six randomised controlled trials (not brilliant, as risk groups formed small minorities) included 800 risk patients. The duration of influenza symptoms was reduced by 1.2 days (95% CI, 0.1–2.2) if Relenza was used (from 6 days to 5). Relenza also reduced the risk of complications requiring antibiotics. No data on hospitalisation were provided.

○ (2001) Comparison of elderly people's technique in using two dry powder inhalers to deliver zanamivir: randomised controlled trial. *BMJ.* **322**: 577–9.
Delivery of zanamivir was as a dry powder through a Diskhaler. The study concluded that most elderly people (i.e. one cohort deemed to be at high risk) were unable to use the inhaler device, so treatment with the drug was unlikely to be effective unless this delivery system could be improved.

● NICE 58 (February 2003): Guidance on the use of zanamivir, oseltamivir and amantidine
These should be used if influenza A or B is circulating in the community, and also in at-risk groups, namely those with chronic respiratory or renal disease, significant cardiovascular disease (not hypertension) or diabetes, the immunocompromised and those over 65 years of age.

Women's health

Hormone replacement therapy

This is ongoing, always topical and problematic. Trials are mainly observational, and are inevitably biased as women who take HRT are likely to be educated and in a higher socio-economic group with better diet, etc. They are also more likely to be compliant. Ethnic-minority patients are less likely than Caucasians to take HRT.

- Around 15% of women aged 45–54 years are taking HRT.

- Around 50% discontinue treatment after the first year.

The target population includes the following:

- hysterectomy and oophorectomy patients under 45 years of age

- women with a history of previous osteoporotic fracture

- women on long-term steroid treatment

- the prematurely menopausal (under 45 years).

You need to decide whether you are starting HRT for symptomatic or preventive reasons.

Advantages

1 *Osteoporosis*: from the menopause, bone mass decreases by 1–3% per year. The lifetime risk of a white female having an osteoporotic fracture is 40%. HRT halves this if it is taken for 10 years (WHO, 1994), and gives an improvement in bone mass of *c*. 5% per year. By comparison, bisphosphonates give an improvement of 4% per year, and calcium supplements (1000 mg/day) give an improvement of 1% per year. Selective oestrogen receptor modulators (SERMs) also have an effect. Thus HRT is not the ultimate solution; you need to consider lifestyle, smoking and alcohol consumption.

   - MORE (Multiple Outcomes of Raloxifene Evaluation trial)

     ○ (2002) *Osteoporos Int.* **13**: 907–13.
       Raloxifene may reduce the vertebral fracture rate by up to 68% in the first year as well as reducing the risk of oestrogen-receptor-positive breast cancer by 80%. SERMs do not improve vasomotor symptoms.

2 *Cerebrovascular disease*: stroke is the third most common cause of death. The Framingham study is the only study to date to show an increase in stroke in postmenopausal women who are oestrogen users. All other studies have shown either no change or a decrease.

- ○ Sherwin *et al.* (1998) *Proc Soc Exp Biol Med.* **217**: 17–22.
  Women who were taking oestrogen fared better with regard to cognitive function than non-users. Other studies have yielded conflicting results.

3 *Diabetes*:

- ○ (2003) *Ann Int Med.* **138**: 1–9.
  This subanalysis of the heart and oestrogen/progestin replacement study (HERS) found that combined HRT may reduce the risk of developing diabetes by a third. The number needed to treat (NNT) is 30.

4 *Alzheimer's disease*:

- ○ (2003) Women's health study. *JAMA.* **289**: 2673–84.
  This study found a two-fold increase in the risk of dementia in women taking combined HRT.

- ○ (2002) *JAMA.* **288**: 2123–9.
  This study found that women who had been taking HRT for 3 years showed a 40% reduction and those who had been taking HRT for 10 years showed a 60% reduction in the likelihood that they would go on to develop the disease.

- ○ (1998) *J Neurol Neurosurg Psychiatry.* **67**: 779–81.
  This case-controlled study of women under 60 years of age showed benefits in HRT users that lasted up to 5 years after stopping HRT.

5 *Colonic cancer*:

- ○ (2003) Women's health study. *JAMA.* **289**: 2673–84.
  This study confirmed work from previous cohorts that HRT reduces the risk of colonic cancer by about one-third.

6 *Leg ulcers*:

- ○ (2002) *Lancet.* **359**: 675–7.
  This study found a 35% reduction in leg ulcers among women who were taking HRT.

Disadvantages

1 *Breast cancer*:

- ○ Beral *et al.* (1997) *Lancet.* **350**: 1047–59.
  This study looked at 52 705 women with breast cancer and 108 411 women without the disease. A total of 51 case-controlled studies highlighted a small increase in the risk of breast cancer in women on long-term HRT. WHI (2002) *JAMA.* **288**: 321–33 and the Million Women Study (2003) *Lancet.* **362**: 419–27 are the two most recent studies giving slightly higher figures.

Time on HRT	Breast cancer at age 50–70 years	Extra breast cancer cases with HRT
never	45/1000	—
5 years	47/1000	2/1000
10 years	51/1000	6/1000
15 years	57/1000	12/1000

The increased risk of breast cancer disappears around 5 years after stopping HRT.

o (2002) *JAMA*. **287**: 735–41.
   Confirmed the link of breast cancer with recent use of HRT. All types of breast cancer were
   doubled in women who had taken HRT for up to 5 years.

o (1999) *JAMA*.
   This and a further study in 2000 showed that women taking HRT who develop breast cancer have
   a better prognosis, are less likely to be node-positive and more likely to be oestrogen-receptor-
   positive.

2 *Coronary heart disease*: around 21% of women die of coronary heart disease and
   the risk increases postmenopausally. By the age of 80 years it is the same as the
   rate for men.

o (2002) *CMO Update*. 33.
   This has confirmed that we should no longer be advising our patients that HRT reduces the risk of
   coronary heart disease.

o (1991) *NEJM*. **325**: 756–62.
   HRT was thought to reduce the risk by 30–50% (although in the first year of taking it there may
   have been a transient increase). This was shown in smokers on HRT for 7 years in the Framingham study, and was confirmed by the nurses' study.

o (2002) The Women's Health Initiative Study. *JAMA*. **288**: 321–33.
   This study of 16 608 women on continuous combined HRT (equine oestrogen and medroxyproges-
   terone acetate, i.e. premique) vs. placebo found that the risks of coronary heart disease, stroke and
   pulmonary embolism were higher than acceptable, and the trial was terminated. There is an
   oestrogen-only arm which is still in progress.

o (2002) Postmenopausal women on HRT and the primary prevention of cardiovascular disease.
   Ann Int Med. **137**: 273–84.
   This meta-analysis of 21 studies reporting the incidence of cardiovascular disease, coronary artery
   disease, stroke and associated mortality found that there was not a significant reduction in the
   relative risk of cardiovascular disease or coronary heart disease. The relative risk of *death* due to
   cardiovascular or coronary heart disease among HRT users showed a small benefit.

o (2003) Relationship between HRT and ischaemic heart disease in women: prospective observational study. *BMJ*. **326**: 426–8.
   This study was based on data from an early study of Danish nurses (19 898 subjects aged over 45
   years). HRT showed no protective effect on ischaemic heart disease. Women with diabetes who
   were taking HRT had an increased risk of ischaemic heart disease and death from all causes.

o (2003) *Br J Gen Pract*. **53**: 191–6.
   This case-controlled study found no evidence that HRT reduced the risk of ischaemic heart disease
   (OR, 1.32; 95% CI, 0.93–1.87).

o (1998) *JAMA*. **280**: 605–13.
   This was a randomised trial of oestrogen plus progesterone for secondary prevention of coronary
   heart disease in postmenopausal women. In 2763 postmenopausal women with coronary heart
   disease, no significant difference in secondary outcomes compared with placebo was found.
     Several studies have shown that women taking HRT have lower LDL- and higher HDL-choles-
   terol levels. A recent Government-funded study has shown that in women taking HRT their risk
   of non-fatal myocardial infarction was reduced by as much as 61%, depending on the HRT
   preparation.

3 *Endometrial cancer*: if the uterus is intact, at least 10 days of progestogen in the cycle of HRT are needed. Even with the use of progestogen there is an increased risk of endometrial cancer (RR = 1.4), albeit only a small risk.

4 *Veno-thromboembolism*:

o (1996) *Lancet*. **348**: 977–80.
   In non-HRT users there were 1 in 10 000 events per year, compared with 3 in 10 000 in HRT users (RR = 2.11–3.9). If the woman is under 40 years of age and has had a previous clot or there is a strong family history, the *Drug and Therapeutics Bulletin* recommends thrombophilic screening prior to starting HRT.

5 *Ovarian cancer*:

o (2002) *JAMA*. **288**: 334–41.
   This study found that women who took oestrogen-only preparations for 10 years or more were at higher risk of developing ovarian cancer (by up to 60%). Women who had had bilateral oophorectomy were excluded from the study.

6 *Cervical cancer*:

o *Eur J Cancer Prev*.
   This study found that stopping long-term combined HRT increased the risk of cervical cancer by at least 50%.

7 *Weight gain*:
   This has not been demonstrated in randomised controlled trials, although bloating can be a temporary side-effect. Khoo *et al.* (1998) *Med J Aust*. **168**: 216–20 found that weight gain at the time of menopause was around 1 stone, whereas with HRT it was around 10 pounds.

Miscellaneous

Estren is a new oestrogen under development, which researchers are confident will not increase the risk of breast cancer.

Alternatives to HRT

The following may help hot flushes:

- phyto-oestrogens (found in chick peas, lentils, soya products, etc.)
  - an HRT cake is available which is rich in phyto-oestrogens
  - there have been several small randomised controlled trials (e.g. comparing soy flour with wheat flour), but they have found no significant reduction in hot flushes
  - other trials have found a reduced severity of flushing, but no change in frequency
  - it is worth noting that hot flushes are rarely reported as a problem in China and Japan (it is open to question whether this is dietary or genetic)
- St John's wort (also used for mood disturbances)
- ginseng

- Mexican yam

- Scisanava, black and blue Cohosh; red clover

- acupuncture.

Menorrhagia

Menorrhagia is the loss of >80 mL of blood (with either regular or irregular menstrual cycles), usually based on a patient's perception. It is important to assess the condition properly for primary and secondary causes.

Around 28% of women feel that menstruation is excessive, and 5% consult their GP.

○ (1999) Medical management of menorrhagia. *BMJ.* **319**: 1343–5.

○ (2001) *Br J Gen Pract.* **52**: 108–13.
   This questionnaire study found that if a woman perceives that the heaviness of her periods is interfering with her life, she is 3.5 times more likely to consult a doctor. It was concluded that quality of life should be focused on by GPs.

In 1998, the Royal College of Obstetricians and Gynaecologists published evidence-based guidelines in favour of using tranexamic acid with or without mefanamic acid to reduce loss (*see* below). They do not recommend routine thyroid function tests, as there is no real evidence-based link.

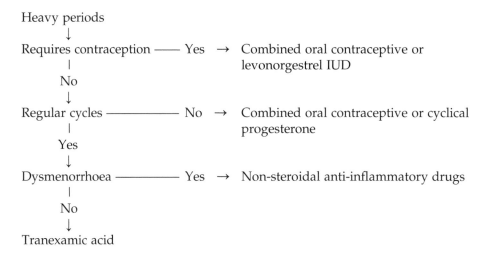

Heavy periods
   ↓
Requires contraception ── Yes → Combined oral contraceptive or
   | levonorgestrel IUD
   No
   ↓
Regular cycles ──────── No → Combined oral contraceptive or cyclical
   | progesterone
   Yes
   ↓
Dysmenorrhoea ───────── Yes → Non-steroidal anti-inflammatory drugs
   |
   No
   ↓
Tranexamic acid

Combined oral contraceptive pill

In the UK, 25% of women aged 16–49 years and 50% of women in their twenties are on the pill.

There are three generations of combined pill.

1 First generation: (e.g. Norinyl-1, Ovran)
- first produced in the 1960s
- high dose of oestrogen (increased veno-thromboembolism (VTE) risk)
- avoided now unless specifically needed.

2 Second generation:
- lower oestrogen
- similar progestogen to first-generation pill.

3 Third generation:
- produced in the 1980s
- lower dose of oestrogen
- new form of progestogen (less androgenic than second-generation products)
- 1995 pill scare – Committee on Safety of Medicines stated that the VTE risk was doubled in users of pills that contained gestodene or desogestrel. This was based on unpublished trials with no confidence intervals. It was the first time that progestogens had been implicated.

Veno-thromboembolism

In 1 year:

- 5 in 100 000 women will develop VTE

- 15 in 100 000 will develop VTE if taking the second-generation pill levonorgestrel/norethisterone

- 25 in 100 000 will develop VTE if taking the third-generation pill gestodene/desogestrel

- 60 in 100 000 will develop VTE in pregnancy.

The absolute risk as opposed to the relative risk is small.

If after 1 year of pill use a woman has not experienced a clot, it is thought that the subsequent risk will then be much lower.

Since the 1980s, the accepted risk for VTE due to combined oral contraceptives has been 30 in 100 000. Therefore studies did not necessarily suggest an increased risk in third-generation pills, but rather a reduced risk and an increased risk with second-generation pills than originally thought.

In 1999, the Department of Health announced an end to the 1995 restrictions on prescribing third-generation pills.

Risk assessment
It is important to assess risk before initiating treatment and at each review.

- VTE increases with increasing age.

- BMI $> 35 \text{ kg/m}^2$ quadruples the risk of VTE. There are other alternatives, so use them.

- Smoking doubles the risk of VTE.

- Family history – first-degree relative under 45 years of age with VTE/primary thrombotic tendency.

- Ask about migraines (focal), breast cancer, pregnancy, undiagnosed vaginal bleeding and diabetes.

- Measure blood pressure.

Latest UK studies

○ (2001) Third-generation oral contraceptives and the risk of venous thrombosis: meta-analysis. *BMJ*. **323**: 131–4.
This meta-analysis supports the view that third-generation pills pose a greater risk than second-generation pills with regard to venous thrombosis. The overall adjusted odds ratio was 1.7 (95% CI, 1.4–2.0). The nine case-control studies looked at patients who had had a thrombosis and whether they used the oral contraceptive pill. This does not prove that the pill caused the clots.

○ Farmer *et al.* (2000) The effects of the 1995 pill scare on VTE rates among COC users. *BMJ*. **321**: 477–9.
In 1995 the Committee on Safety of Medicines based their advice on unpublished studies with no confidence intervals. The above study showed no change in the incidence of VTE since the pill scare, despite a decrease in prescribing third-generation pills from 53.4% to 14%. Therefore the findings are not consistent with third-generation oral contraceptives doubling the rate of VTE! A further study has confirmed these findings.

○ Farmer *et al.* (2000) A comparison of the risks of venous thromboembolic disease in association with different combined oral contraceptives. *Br J Clin Pharmacol*. **49**: 580–90.
No significant difference was found between second- and third-generation pills. Obesity is an important risk factor for women on the pill. BMI > 35 kg/m^2 increases the risk of VTE by fourfold, and BMI in the range 30–35 kg/m^2 doubles the risk. Smoking was found to be a significant risk factor in this study, doubling the risk of VTE.

○ (1999) Mortality associated with oral contraceptive use: 25-year follow-up of 46 000 women from the RCGP oral contraceptive study. *BMJ*. **318**: 96–100.
Among a total of 1599 deaths reported from 1400 practices in the UK, 945 deaths were of women who had at some time used the pill, and 654 deaths were of non-users. The death rate from all causes combined was 21% lower than in the UK population (for age). This finding was not unexpected, as women with severe chronic illnesses were excluded. Most of the effects on mortality occurred in current or recent users, and few if any effects persisted after stopping use for 10 years.

The following findings have been confirmed.

- The risk of breast cancer is slightly increased, but there is no excess risk after stopping for more than 10 years.

○ (2002) *NEJM*. **346**: 2025–32.

- The risk of cervical cancer is increased, but there is no excess risk after stopping for 10 years. There is a question as to whether the combined oral contraceptive pill potentiates human papilloma virus, rather than the latter reflecting promiscuity.

○ (2002) *Lancet*. **359**: 1085–92.

○ (2002) *Lancet*. **359**: 1093–101.
These studies found that women who had taken the combined oral contraceptive pill for 5–9 years were nearly three times more likely than non-users to develop cervical cancer. Women who had taken the pill for more than 10 years were four times more likely to develop cervical cancer.

○ (2003) *Lancet*. **361**: 1159–67.
This systematic review of cervical cancer and use of hormonal contraceptives looked at 28 eligible studies.

• The risk of circulatory disease is increased in users/recent users of the pill.

• The risk of ovarian cancer is *reduced* in users/recent users of the pill.

Implanon

This was launched in September 1999 (following problems with Norplant relating to the insertion and removal of six rods).

It consists of a single semi-rigid rod of dimensions 40 mm × 2 mm. Insertion should be performed subdermally, and the device releases 30–40 µg of etonogestrel per day. It lasts for 3 years.

Amenorrhoea is reported in 21% of users, and irregular bleeding is problematic (as always with progestogen-only methods) in 17% of women.

There have been reports of fractures of the implant following minor trauma.

Coils

1 Mirena:
    • licensed for 5 years only (even if fitted in women over 40 years), although it is probably OK for 7 years
    • causes atrophy of the endometrium
    • most women ovulate only occasionally after first year of use.

2 Gynefix:
    • frameless IUD consisting of six copper tubes on a nylon thread, knotted at one end, that anchors into the uterine fundus
    • failure rate is <1% for up to 5 years of use
    • expulsion rate is low.

3 T-Safe 380:
    • easy to insert, even in nulliparous women (compared with Multiload 375)
    • since Ortho-Gynae T380 was withdrawn (for commercial reasons), it has been a good option
    • licensed for 8 years (10 years on a named patient basis).

4 Nova T 380:
    • slimline for insertion (suitable for nulliparous women or where problems are anticipated)

- failure rate at 2 years is 1.6 per 100 women; 60% were due to recognised expulsion.

At least 300 mm of copper is needed for contraception to be effective.

Other contraceptives

1 *Eva patch* (norelgestromin and ethinyloestradiol; Cilest through the skin). This is worn for 3 out of 4 weeks; have break through bleeding (need to change patch weekly). Recent studies show that it is as effective as the combined oral contraceptive pill.

2 *Yasmin* (drospirenone)

   o (2002) *Drug Ther Bull.* **40**: 57–9.
      There is a small loss of weight initially, which is then regained. The risk of deep vein thrombosis is probably increased fourfold (compared with levonorgestrel) (similar risk to Dianette).

3 *Nuvaring* (120 µg efonogestrel and 15 µg oestrogen). This is worn for 3 out of 4 weeks. Have BTB.

4 *Cerazette* is a 75 µg desogestrel progestogen-only pill (but the manufacturer has applied for a licence for a 12-hour window). It inhibits ovulation in 97% of cases, and is a good option for younger women.

5 *Nesterone* in the following different forms is going through trials (it is not active orally):
   - 2-year implant
   - intrauterine system – smaller than Mirena
   - transdermal patch and gel
   - ring (both combined and progestogen only).

Emergency contraception

Around 12% of patients who require emergency contraception are under 16 years of age. Emergency contraception is available free on prescription from GPs, from family planning clinics, youth clinics, walk-in centres, genito-urinary clinics and some Accident and Emergency departments.

o (2003) *J Fam Plan Reprod Health Care.* **29**: 9–16.
   This article contains comprehensive guidance on emergency contraception.

o (1998) *Lancet.* **352**: 428–33.
   A WHO Taskforce randomised controlled trial compared PC4 and levonorgestrel in almost 2000 women from 14 countries. The failure rates were 3.2% and 1.1% for Yupze (PC4) and levonorgestrel, respectively. Identical results were obtained after adjusting for the cycle day on which intercourse took place, BMI and reason for requesting emergency contraception. The side-effects profile was better for levonorgestrel than for PC4.

Although it has taken time, levonelle is now first line, although PC4 is still available. Levonelle has been available over the counter since January 2001 (it is rather expensive, at £20+). This was after pilot studies that showed a high demand and also confirmed that patients were using the drug appropriately and that it was safe.

○ (2002) *Lancet*. **360**: 1803–10.
  This study of 4071 women found that 10 mg of mifeprostone, 1.5 mg of levonorgestrel or two doses of 750 μg levonorgestrel all had similar efficacy in preventing pregnancy.

If a patient weighs over 70 kg, the Oxford Family Planning Association study has confirmed a higher failure rate of the progestogen-only pill. It is advised that patients take 2 × 750 μg followed by 1 × 750 μg levonelle. This also follows for women on enzyme-inducing drugs but is not evidence based. Women should be warned of the greater risk of ectopic pregnancy following emergency contraception.

Other options

Don't forget the IUD can be used up to 5 days after unprotected intercourse (i.e. up to day 19 of a regular 28-day cycle). Medicolegally this is not procuring an abortion (it has been tested in the courts).

○ (2002) Improving teenagers' knowledge of contraception: cluster RCT of teacher-led intervention. *BMJ*. **324**: 1179–83.
  This study found that teachers giving a single lesson on emergency contraception to year 10 pupils improved the number of boys and girls who knew the correct time limits for both types of emergency contraception. It did not change sexual activity or use of emergency contraception.

○ (2002) Young women's accounts of factors influencing their use and non-use of emergency contraception: in-depth interview study. *BMJ*. **325**: 1393–6.
  This study found that the concerns of young women, especially those from deprived inner-city areas, may render them less willing and able to obtain emergency contraception. They find it difficult to ask.

Teenage pregnancies

- Teenagers represent 10% of the population.
- Around 30 in 1000 pregnancies are teenage pregnancies.
- Teenage pregnancies are by definition high risk.
- Around 35% result in termination of pregnancy.
- The UK has the highest teenage pregnancy rate in western Europe.
- Around 93% of teenagers who became pregnant have accessed primary care during the year before conception (compared with 83% of controls).

Health of the Nation 1990

This initiative increased priorities for under-16s, and aimed to halve the rate of teenage pregnancies by 2000. This goal was not met for a number of reasons, including the fact that GPs have little influence on risk-taking behaviour.

Issues relating to teenage pregnancies

1 *Provision of health and sex education.* Teenagers are often unaware of how to obtain contraceptive advice and believe that they have to be over 16 years of age to obtain treatment. However, since the Gillick ruling of October 1985 (now the Fraser guidelines, *see* page 183), this is no longer the case. Teenagers are often willing to run the risk of sexually transmitted diseases and pregnancy, as they think their parents will find out if they see their GP (confidentiality is needed at all levels).

2 *Contraceptive services need to be accessible.* This includes the GP/family planning services/school nurse.

3 *Role of schools.* This includes sex education/behavioural interventions, as well as the need to develop communication skills and sustain the truth that virginity still prevails among the majority (apparently).

○ (2000) GP opportunities for teenage health promotion. *Br J Gen Pract*. **50**: 581.

Modernising Health and Social Services, 2000/01 to 2002/03

This highlights the tackling of teenage pregnancies in the light of the *Health of the Nation* findings, especially prevention of conception and giving support to teenage parents.

○ (2002) *J Health Econ.* **21**: 207–25.
This study showed that policy to improve access to family planning services for under-16s was not reducing pregnancy rates and could increase conception rates. The data were confirmed by the Office of National Statistics.

○ (2002) Interventions to reduce unintended pregnancies among adolescents: systematic review. *BMJ.* **324**: 1426–30.
This study concluded that primary prevention strategies to date do not delay initiation of sexual intercourse, improve use of birth control or reduce the number of teenage pregnancies.

○ (2002) Young people's and professionals' views about ways to reduce teenage pregnancy rates: to agree or not to agree. *Fam Plan Reprod Health Care.* **28**: 85–90.
This study showed that professionals favoured young people's services, while young people emphasised the need for young-person-centred services.

Chlamydia

- The prevalence of chlamydia is 1–29% (Chief Medical Officer's report, 1998, probably underestimated).

- Reported rates are 800 in 100 000 in 15 to 19-year-olds.

- Around 70% of women and 50% of men are asymptomatic, but there may be non-specific symptoms.

- The cost to the NHS is £50 million per year.

- It is the most common curable bacterial sexually transmitted disease in Europe.

- It is the most common cause of pelvic inflammatory disease (hence issues of ectopics, infertility and litigation).

- High-risk groups include the following:
  - terminations of pregnancy
  - 16 to 25-year-olds
  - little is known about the male population.

- Behavioural risk factors include the following:
  - multiple partners
  - single marital status
  - ethnicity
  - low school-leaving age.

  ○ (1998) Chief Medical Officer's Report 1998. *BMJ*. **316**: 351.
  This recommended opportunistic screening of the following:
  - sexually active women under 25 years of age
  - older women with a new partner or two or more partners in the last year.
  The report recommended opportunistic screening for chlamydia and to consider testing on clinical grounds the genito-urinary clinic setting, termination of pregnancy and high-risk groups prior to instrumentation (including IUCDs).

Pilot study in progress for screening in primary care

The aim is to assess the feasibility and accessibility of opportunistic screening using the ligase chain reaction on a first-catch urine sample (more acceptable than swabs!). The objective is to estimate true costs, and to determine the health benefits, accessibility and cost-effectiveness of screening.

The choice of test is as follows:

- enzyme-linked immunosorbent assay (ELISA)

- polymerase chain reaction (PCR)

- ligase chain reaction (LCR).

ELISA has a sensitivity of 60–70% and a low specificty (i.e. would lead to missed cases and a high proportion of false positives). Both PCR and LCR have a sensitivity of 80–90% and a specificity of 99%.

  ○ (2002) Pilot study to assess the presence of *Chlamydia trachomatis* in urine from 18 to 30-year-old males using enzyme immunoassay/immunofluorescence and PCR. *J Fam Reprod Health Care*. **28**: 36–7.
  Enzyme immunoassay and immunofluorescence were positive for 12/71 (17%) cases. There was reduced sensitivity compared with PCR which was positive for a further 15/71 (21%), giving a yield of 38% (this is more expensive than enzyme immunoassay/immunofluorescence). Most previous research has been done with females. This study shows a significant yield of positive results in young males which could be tested opportunistically.

Screening

The first phase of the screening programme is now under way in 10 locations following the success of the pilot studies.

Evidence for the effectiveness of screening for *Chlamydia*

○ (1996) Prevention of PID by screening for *Chlamydia*. *NEJM*. **334**: 1362–6.

○ (1993) *Sex Transm Dis*.
A randomised controlled trial and several case studies have all shown that screening significantly reduces the prevalence of genito-urinary infections and pelvic inflammatory disease in women.

○ (1998) The case for screening. *BMJ*. **316**: 1474.

○ (1999) *Br J Gen Pract*. **49**: 455.
The first of these two studies looked at the effectiveness of home screening, and the second confirmed that there was a good uptake (83%) with postal samples.

Screening implications for GPs

1 Extra time needed:
- samples from at-risk patients
- training for practice staff
- sexual history from all female patients
- pre-test counselling
- counselling for patients who test positive
- partner notification and treatment
- ensuring compliance with and follow-up of treatment.

2 Extra resources needed:
- staff training
- laboratory tests.

3 Public health:
- little is known publicly
- in 1997, 26% of 16- to 24-year-olds had heard of chlamydia
- the screening programme would have to involve the media.

4 Issues:
- compliance – requires sexual abstinence
- contact tracing (6-month history)
- consider test of cure
- genito-urinary referral – confidentiality issue/insurance forms, etc.

○ (2001) Qualitative analysis of psychososcial impact of diagnosis of C. *trachomatis*: implications for screening. *BMJ*. **322**: 195–9.
This study identified three areas of concern for women after diagnosis of chlamydia, namely the stigma associated with sexually transmitted diseases, their future reproductive health and informing current partners. It concluded that messages accompanying screening should not imply that diagnosis and treatment will not prevent infertility. Furthermore, it suggested that information given to women before screening should seek to normalise and destigmatise chlamydia infection, in order to reduce the negative psychosocial impact of a positive diagnosis.

Single vs. multiple dose regimens

○ (1996) *Bandolier*. **28**: 4–6.
This meta-analysis of short-term randomised controlled trials indicated that single-dose azithromycin may be as effective as a 7-day course of doxycycline. More information is needed.

One systematic review of randomised controlled trials in pregnant women (Cochrane Library, 1999) showed that single-dose azithromycin is as effective as 7 days of erythromycin. However, the effects of azithromycin in pregnancy have not been extensively studied.

Pre-menstrual syndrome

This is a distinct disorder that occurs in the luteal phase of the cycle due to release of progesterone triggered by ovulation. There is no evidence of hormonal imbalance, despite the popularity of the progesterone deficiency theory. Meta-analyses have confirmed that progesterone products are no more effective than placebo.

There is no diagnostic test. The best way to diagnose premensstrual syndrome (PMS) is by asking the patient to keep a 3-month diary which should show cyclical premenstrual deterioration with postmenstrual cure.

Treatment

There are two broad approaches.

Suppressing ovulation

- Combined oral contraceptive pill (variable response).

- Danazol (several randomised controlled trials prove benefit; long-term use is limited due to the masculinising effects of the drug).

- Oestrogen patches or implants – progestogenic endometrial protection (e.g. Mirena) is needed, as well as assessment of the endometrium at the outset so as not to risk falsely reassuring the woman that bleeding is normal if she has endometrial cancer.

- Gonadotropin-releasing hormone (GnRH) (pharmacological menopause – time limited unless add-back HRT or tibolone is used).

- Oophorectomy (rarely justified).

Changing serotonin status

- Vitamin B_6 (50–100 mg maximum, as there is a risk of peripheral neuropathy)

○ (1999) Systematic review. *BMJ*. **318**: 1375–81.
The conclusions of this review were limited due to the 'low quality' of most trials, but there were trends towards positive efficacy.

- Selective serotonin reuptake inhibitors (SSRIs) appear to be seven times more effective than placebo, but must not be prescribed with St John's wort.

Other issues

Agnus castus fruit extract

o (2001) *BMJ*. **322**: 134–7.
  This was traditionally used to relieve PMS. In this study of 178 German women who were randomised for three cycles, *Agnus castus* fruit was found to be significantly more effective than placebo. It appears to be safe.

Progesterone and progestogens

o (2001) *BMJ*. **323**: 776–80.
  This systematic review found no evidence to support the use of progesterone and progestogens in PMS.

Breast cancer

This accounted for 27% of all female cancers in 1995. It is the most common female cancer, and it is the cause of 18% of all female deaths.

Around 5% of all breast cancers are linked to specific single gene defects, 80% of which are due to BRCA 1 or 2.

Breast screening

The NHS breast screening programme was introduced in England and Wales in 1988 on the recommendation of the Forrest Committee. In 1992, the Department of Health set a target for a reduction in breast cancer mortality of 25% by 2000 in 55- to 69-year-olds. It is currently estimated that 1250 lives are saved each year by the screening programme. However, a Danish study disputes this.

o (2001) Cochrane review on screening for breast cancer with mammography. *Lancet*. **358**: 1340–2.
  There is no evidence that clinical examination, breast ultrasonography or teaching self-examination are effective in increasing early detection of breast cancer.

The Leningrad and Shanghai studies are large randomised controlled trials that failed to demonstrate a reduction in mortality from breast cancer or increased detection by teaching self-examination.

Mammography has been shown in a Swedish randomised controlled trial to reduce mortality by up to 40%, the benefit being greatest in those aged 50–70 years. At present it is the best screening tool available. Compared with symptomatic breast cancers, screen-detected cancers are smaller and more likely to be non-invasive. If they are invasive, they are more likely to be better differentiated and node-negative.

○ (2002) Long-term effects of mammography screening. *Lancet.* **359**: 909–19.
   This meta-analysis of four Swedish randomised controlled trials showed that women aged 55–69 years showed a 21% reduction in breast cancer mortality if invited for screening.

It has been calculated that for every 2 million women screened, one extra cancer after 10 years may be caused by the radiation delivered to the breast during mammography.

No increase in anxiety has been found in women invited to attend for screening, unless there is a need for recall.

HRT reduces the sensitivity of mammography (from 77% to 65%) and is associated with more false positives.

○ (2000) Effect of NHS Breast Screening Programme on mortality from breast cancer in England and Wales, 1990-98: comparison of observed with predicted mortality. *BMJ.* **321**: 665–9.
   This study showed that in women aged 40–79 years, since 1991 there has been a 21% decrease in mortality (6% due to screening and 15% due to treatment).

○ (2000) *BMJ.* **321**: 647–8.
   This covering editorial discusses factors other than mortality that determine the success of a screening programme.

Since the above study there have been various criticisms in terms of not reflecting true data. For example, if a patient has received radiotherapy and goes on to develop heart failure and die, this would be recorded as a cardiovascular death. In reality, such numbers would be small, but further studies are needed.

○ (2002) *Lancet.* **360**: 817–24.
   This study has shown that tamoxifen given to *healthy women* at high risk reduces the risk of breast cancer by a third over 4 years. There was an increased risk of veno-thromboembolism.

Cervical cancer

• The incidence of cervical cancer in the UK is 10 per 100 000.

• The mortality rate is 5 per 100 000.

• The incidence of the disease peaks at 30–35 and 70–75 years of age.

• Around 95% of cervical cancers are squamous cell and 5% are adenocarcinomas.

• The most important risk factor is human papilloma virus (HPV).

Cervical screening

• Current screening is performed every 3 to 5 years. Around 83% of women aged 25–64 years have been screened.

• Abnormal changes graded as CIN 1 should have a repeat at 3 months.

• If the smear is persistently abnormal, colposcopy should be performed.

• Women with smears graded as CIN 2 or 3 should have colposcopy performed.

Liquid-based cytology combined with HPV screening

- The first pilot study is now complete.

- It shows a reduced need for repeats from 10% to 0.5%.

- The 18-month pilot involved 12 655 samples.

- The cost is £4.75 per test compared with £1 for a PAP smear. However, it is argued that the technique is economical as there is a reduced need for repeats.

- HPV genotype/DNA screening is used to separate women with borderline smears into high- and low-risk groups, especially those over 30 years of age.

  ○ (2001) *BMJ*. **322**: 893–4.

  ○ (2003) Cross-sectional study of conventional cervical smears, monolayer cytology and human papilloma virus DNA testing for cervical screening. *BMJ*. **326**: 733–6.
    In this study the three techniques were compared simultaneously. The results supported conventional screening, as the other tests were no better, and the monolayer cytology was less reliable.

Computer screening
PAPNET is a software package designed to avoid 'human error' in interpreting cytology.

  ○ (1999) *Lancet*. **253**: 1382.
    This study concluded that the technique was more accurate, quicker and cheaper.

Cervical cancer vaccine

This has been around for several years now. There are two trials ongoing in the UK and the USA, the results of which are awaited.

Ovarian cancer

- The incidence in the UK is 20 per 100 000 (and it appears to be increasing).

- The mortality rate is 15 per 100 000.

- Women with the BRCA 1 gene have a 50% lifetime risk, and those with the BRCA 2 gene have a 30% lifetime risk.

Ovarian screening

There is no proven role for screening, but methods would include Ca125 and transvaginal ultrasound scanning. In some areas, women with one or more first-degree relatives with ovarian cancer may be offered yearly Ca125 and ultrasound scan. They should be made aware of the limitations of these mthods and the lack of evidence for their effectiveness.

The Medical Research Council has launched a 10-year trial (UK Collaborative Trial of Ovarian Cancer Screening) of 200 000 postmenopausal women, looking at transvaginal vs. Ca125 on a yearly basis to try to establish the effectiveness of these methods in terms of their impact on mortality/morbidity and cost.

Antenatal care

Down's syndrome screening

Down's syndrome is the most common chromosomal abnormality at birth. Its incidence is related to maternal age.

Chief Medical Officer's Update 31 (October 2001)

On 30 April 2001, the Government announced a Down's syndrome screening programme as part of antenatal modernisation. The test should consist of at least a double test, namely alphafetoprotein (AFP) and human chorionic gonadotropin (HCG), but it would be preferable to move to a triple test (AFP, HCG and unconjugated oestradiol) or even a quadruple one (AFP, HCG, unconjugated oestradiol and inhibin A; costs around £22) in the second trimester.

One of these should be available to all women by 2004.

○ (2002) Retrospective audit of different antenatal screening policies for Down's syndrome in eight district general hospitals in one health region. *BMJ*. **325**: 15–17.
These audit results showed that serum screening for Down's syndrome did not improve detection rates or reduce the number of cases needing amniocentesis. Thus serum and nuchal translucency screening may be less advantageous than was previously thought.

○ (2001) Screening for Down's syndrome: effects, safety and cost-effectiveness on first- and second-trimester strategies. *BMJ*. **323**: 423–5.
This study compared nine strategies for screening currently available in the UK, looking at 10 000 women in 1995. It concluded that the choice should be between the integrated test (first-trimester nuchal translucency, pregnancy-associated plasma protein A (PAPP-A) and second-trimester quadruple test), the first-trimester combined test (nuchal translucency, PAPP-A and HCG), the quadruple test or nuchal translucency measurements, depending on how much service providers are willing to pay and the total budget available.

Nuchal scanning as screening for Down's syndrome

○ (1998) *Lancet*. **352**: 337–8.
This study of 96 000 women found a detection rate of 80% when nuchal scanning was performed at 10–14 weeks. The detection rate for the triple test is 60%. Although this appears to be worse, the triple test is done in the second trimester, and article reviewers have pointed out that up to 40% of trisomy 21 foetuses will die at between 10 and 14 weeks, so the figures are probably not comparable.

○ (2001) *Lancet*. **358**: 1665–8.
This study looked at nasal bones on ultrasound scans in foetuses at 11–14 weeks' gestation. Around 73% of foetuses affected by Down's syndrome had no nasal bones, compared with 0.5% of normal foetuses. This finding will have implications for future screening.

○ (2003) Antenatal screening for Down's with the quadruple test. *Lancet*. **361**: 835–6.
This study found that the quadruple test detected 81% of Down's syndrome pregnancies. This calculation used maternal age and four markers, and concluded that it should be the test of choice.

Since March 2001, all NHS regions should have had a Down's syndrome co-ordinator in post, and by 2004 each hospital should have a local co-ordinator to develop services and offer support to GPs, midwives and pregnant women.

The UK National Screening Committee is developing national standards for screening and counselling for parents who find out that they are carrying a child with Down's syndrome.

HIV testing

- Around 300 babies each year are born with HIV (mainly in London).

- Up to 80% of these cases could be prevented by the use of antiviral drugs, lower segment Caesarean section and avoiding breastfeeding.

Women are now being offered HIV screening at booking, especially in high-risk areas, to reduce the risk of transmission (national targets were adopted in 1999). Although screening is offered, there is not always the necessary counselling (GUM style) to explain fully the implications of a positive test. Are mothers consenting to a test without being fully informed? Does this matter?

○ (2001) Antenatal detection of HIV: national surveillance and unlinked anonymous survey. *BMJ.* **323**: 376–7.
This study compared data from 1997 with data from 1999, and showed an increase in the number of HIV-infected mothers detected (both before and during pregnancy). It also showed a reduction in the estimated number of babies who acquired HIV from their mothers.

Pre-eclampsia

This condition complicates around 10% of pregnancies. It is believed that antiplatelets may have a role in prophylaxis, but there is much conflicting evidence.

The CLASP trial and subsequent meta-analyses showed no benefit. However, the use of aspirin in women at high risk of early-onset pre-eclampsia may be beneficial.

○ (2001) *BMJ.* **322**: 329.
This systematic review of 39 trials involving more than 30 000 women showed that antiplatelets reduced the development of pre-eclampsia toxaemia by 15%. It concluded that aspirin should be started before 12 weeks, *but* there is a high number needed to treat. Women should be given the option of deciding.

○ (2002) The relationship between maternal work, ambulatory blood pressure and pregnancy hypertension. *J Epidemiol Commun Health.* **56**: 389–93.
This study of primiparous women in midtrimester (working status unknown), in which other factors (age, smoking, BMI, marital status) were adjusted for, found that blood pressure readings were higher in working women. These women were almost five times more likely to go on to develop pre-eclampsia.

Research in the USA has shown that there may be a window in the first trimester for detection of pre-eclampsia using sex-hormone-binding globulin as a marker. This is not currently used.

Borderline iron-deficiency anaemia

The WHO definition of anaemia in pregnancy is a haemoglobin concentration of less than 11 g/dL. There are four Cochrane Reviews on the subject.

Iron and folate supplementation prevents low haemoglobin levels at birth, but there is no evidence that this conclusively improves maternal or foetal outcome. At the same time, there is no evidence against supplementation (i.e. no definitive conclusion!).

Postnatal depression

○ (2000) *Drug Ther Bull.* **38**: 33–7.

• One in 10 women become depressed after childbirth (70 000 women/year).

• Around 50% are still having problems 6 months postnatally.

• This is different from 'baby blues', which are common around days 3–5 (up to day 10), do not require treatment, and are less severe than puerperal psychosis.

• Postnatal depression tends to start around weeks 4–6.

• It is important to diagnose and treat this condition early in order to minimise problems with bonding within the family.

Edinburgh Postnatal Depression Scale

○ (1987) *Br J Psychiatry.* **150**: 782–6.
This scale was developed in primary care to improve detection by screening. It is used at 6–8 weeks postnatally and is scored by a health professional (GP, health visitor or midwife).

1	I have been able to laugh and see the funny side of things.	
	As much as I always could	0
	Not quite so much now	1
	Definitely not so much now	2
	Not at all	3
2	I have looked forward with enjoyment to things.	
	As much as I ever did	0
	Rather less than I used to	1
	Definitely less than I used to	2
	Hardly at all	3
3	I have blamed myself unnecessarily when things went wrong.	
	Yes, most of the time	3
	Yes, some of the time	2
	Not very often	1
	No, never	0
4	I have been anxious or worried for no good reason.	
	No, not at all	0
	Hardly ever	1
	Yes, sometimes	2
	Yes, very often	3

  5   I have felt scared or panicky for no good reason.
       Yes, quite a lot   3
       Yes, sometimes   2
       No, not much   1
       No, not at all   0
  6   Things have been getting on top of me.
       Yes, most of the time I haven't been able to cope at all   3
       Yes, sometimes I haven't been coping as well as usual   2
       No, most of the time I have coped quite well   1
       No, I have been coping as well as ever   0
  7   I have been so unhappy that I have had difficulty sleeping.
       Yes, most of the time   3
       Yes, sometimes   2
       Not very often   1
       No, not at all   0
  8   I have felt sad or miserable.
       Yes, most of the time   3
       Yes, quite often   2
       Not very often   1
       No, not at all   0
  9   I have been so unhappy that I have been crying.
       Yes, most of the time   3
       Yes, quite often   2
       Only occasionally   1
       No, never   0
  10   The thought of harming myself has occurred to me.
       Yes, quite often   3
       Sometimes   2
       Hardly ever   1
       Never   0

Calculate the total score. Of those with scores >13, 92.3% are likely to be suffering from depressive illness. However, the score should not override clinical judgement.

Treatment of postnatal depression

Treatment of proven benefit includes cognitive behavioural therapy, and counselling by a health visitor. SSRIs and tricyclic antidepressants also appear to be safe in breastfeeding women.

There is no evidence to support hormonal treatment, although there is ongoing research into the use of oestrogen (contraindicated in breastfeeding).

○ (2001) Cohort study of depressed mood during pregnancy and after childbirth. *BMJ*. **323**: 257–60.
  This study of 12 059 women in Avon used the Edinburgh Postnatal Depression questionnaire both antenatally, at 18 and 32 weeks' gestation, and postnatally, at 8 weeks and 8 months after the birth. The study concluded that depressive symptoms were not more common or severe after childbirth than during pregnancy. The authors planned to validate and test the hypothesis that childbirth may be a non-specific stressor for depression in most women, and a specific stressor in a subgroup of women, by following mothers through their next pregnancy.

The consequences of screening for and recognising antenatal depression need to be explored in terms of morbidity, treatment and outcome.

Confidential Inquiry into Maternal Deaths, 1997–1999
This found a small reduction in the number of deaths from obstetric causes. However, there was an increase in the number of deaths in women who had concurrent medical or psychological problems. The leading cause of death was suicide during the postnatal period.

Identification of postnatal depression
Thyroperoxidase antibodies, a marker for hypothyroidism, have also been found to be an indicator for postnatal depression when present in early pregnancy.

Men's health

A whole issue of the *British Medical Journal* was dedicated to men's health (3 November 2001). Several studies have shown that men seek help for a given illness later than women. Although they do care about health issues, they find it more difficult to express their fears.

Prostate cancer

www.doh.gov.uk/cancer/prostate.htm

- Around 20 000 new cases are diagnosed each year (second most common male cancer).

- Screening has increased the epidemiological incidence of the disease.

  ○ (2002) *J Natl Cancer Inst.* **94**: 981–90.

- Around 60% of cases have metastatic disease at the time of diagnosis.

  ○ (2001) Screening for prostate cancer in the UK. *BMJ.* **323**: 763–4.
    This is a controversial issue, and systematic reviews have found insufficient evidence to recommend screening. There is no evidence for treatment decisions in the early stages of the disease. Therefore screening may cause more harm than good.

Current UK Government policy (NHS Prostate Cancer Risk Management Programme) confirms the above, but adds that any man can have a prostrate-specific antigen (PSA) test if he wants. Thus screening may creep in, although the test does not satisfy the criteria for a screening programme.

In Stirling, 1627 men aged 40–79 years were screened, and 17 cases of prostate cancer were discovered.

  ○ (2002) Why men with prostate cancer want wider access to PSA testing: qualitative study. *BMJ.* **325**: 737–9.
    This UK study of 52 men with prostate cancer found that most wanted screening, as it would encourage men to be tested (which constitutes responsible health behaviour). They also believed that knowing the diagnosis would reduce mortality, improve quality of life and save the NHS money.

  ○ (2002) Natural experiment examining the impact of aggressive screening and treatment on prostate cancer mortality in two fixed cohorts from Seattle and Connecticut. *BMJ.* **325**: 740–3.

This study looked at 215521 men over a period of 11 years and found no difference in mortality. The trial is ongoing.

○ (2002) *NEJM.* **347**: 781–9.
This study looked at radical prostatectomy vs. watchful waiting in 695 men over a period of 6.2 years. There was no difference in survival rates between the two groups.

○ (2002) *J Clin Epidemiol.* **55**: 603.
This study looked at 1000 men over 50 years of age with prostate cancer. Half of them had been screened with PSA with or without rectal examination. Screening did not improve survival in men under 70 years of age. This supports the view that mass screening should not be introduced.

○ (2001) *Mayo Clin Proc.* **76**: 571–2, 576–81.
This study looked at the doubling time of PSA. A short doubling time was associated with systemic recurrence, whereas a long doubling time was associated with local recurrence.

Measuring the free/total PSA ratio may double the detection rate of prostate cancer (currently the total PSA is used). These findings were reported by the European Urology Association in 2002. The UK National Screening Committee is currently considering this. A genetic test is also being developed in Holland.

Prostate cancer vaccine

This induces antibody production to central metastatic disease. It is currently undergoing clinical trials.

Benign prostatic hypertrophy

- Around 3.3 million men in the UK have benign prostatic hypertrophy (BPH).

- The prime concern in management, besides symptom control, is to ensure that those men who have outflow obstruction do not go on to develop renal failure.

The International Prostate Symptom Score (IPSS) is one way of assessing symptoms over time with treatment.
    The BPH Impact Index is a way of assessing how troublesome the symptoms are.

○ (2001) *Eur Urol.* **40**: 256–63.

Management

1 *Alpha-blockers* (e.g. prazosin, indoramin). These relax the smooth muscle of the prostate. In randomised controlled trials they proved more effective than placebo. They usually produce an improvement within 2–3 weeks. If there is no improvement within 3–4 months, an alternative should be tried.

2 *5-alpha-reductase inhibitors* (e.g. finasteride). These inhibit 5-alpha-reductase, which converts testosterone to dihydroxytestosterone (DHT), that is known to influence prostate growth. Randomised controlled trials have confirmed that

they are more effective than placebo. They cause hyperplasia to regress over 3–6 months (allow 12 months for maximum effect), so are especially suitable if the prostate is very enlarged.

○ (1998) PLESS (Proscar Long-term Efficacy and Safety Study). *NEJM*. **338**: 557–63.
This 4-year randomised controlled trial showed that Proscar improved symptoms, reduced acute retention (57%, NNT = 27) and reduced the need for surgery (55%, NNT = 18). Side-effects included increased hair count in balding men (1553 men in a randomised controlled trial), and in fact the drug is now licensed for this use.

3 *Plant extracts.*
  ● Saw palmetto (*Serona repens*) (Permixon). This is an extract from a cactus-like plant. It has shown success (although the trial did not use a placebo arm). It works in a similar manner to finasteride, and is available over the counter.
  ● β-sitosterol. Trials have shown that this is more effective than placebo in the short term. Side-effects include gastrointestinal symptoms and impotence.
  ● Rye grass pollen extract. It has been suggested that this is beneficial, but trials are as yet inconclusive.

Erectile dysfunction

UK management guidelines for erectile dysfunction were published in 2000.

○ (2000) *BMJ*. **321**: 499–503.
This condition affects up to 52% of men aged 40–70 years. Around 20% have complete erectile failure. It is important to remember to exclude underlying medical problems (e.g. cardiovascular disease, diabetes, depression, smoking) and to check the prostate for the sake of completeness.

If there is a normal libido and secondary sexual characteristics, it is unusual to find a low testosterone level. If sex-hormone-binding globulin (SHBG) and testosterone levels are requested, a ratio can then be determined (i.e. the availability of testosterone).

Treatment

Involve the partner as well as the patient wherever possible.

Sildenafil (Viagra)
This is a selective inhibitor of phosphodiesterase type 5. The best responders are those with psychogenic causes, although the behaviourist approach of Masters and Johnson may be more appropriate.

○ (1998) *NEJM*. **338**: 1397–404.
In six randomised controlled trials, sildenafil was effective and well tolerated compared with placebo.

○ (2001) *J Urol*. **166**: 927–31.
This study found that sildenafil may stop working for many patients after 2 years.

Patients who received an NHS prescription before 14 September 1998 can continue to receive erectile dysfunction treatment (not just the first method they were prescribed) on the NHS (the script should be endorsed 'SLS'). Otherwise, treatment is only available on the NHS for patients with certain medical problems (*see* MIMS or *British National Formulary*), such as prostate cancer, diabetes, spinal cord injury, Parkinson's disease, multiple sclerosis, etc. (12 in total). Private scripts can be written for those who are not eligible for NHS treatment (note that it is cheaper to buy four 100 mg tablets and take half a tablet).

Tadalafil (Cialis)
This drug has a 24-hour action (taken 30 minutes to 12 hours before intercourse). It has been found to improve erection in up to 81% of men (on the maximum dose), with 75% of intercourse attempts being successful.

Apomorphine (Uprima) (dopamine-receptor agonist)
This drug has been licensed for erectile dysfunction. Currently there are no prescribing restrictions. There is a 1 in 500 risk of syncope due to vasovagal response, so care is needed with the first dose and when increasing from 2 to 3 mg.

Intracavernous prostaglandin E_1 (Alprostadil)
Around 80% of men have a satisfactory erection with this drug, but they need to be taught to self-inject.

Intraurethral prostaglandin E_1
The Muse system of pellets is used. Around 30% of men report some discomfort after use. This can cause discontinuation of treatment. One randomised controlled trial showed a satisfactory effect in 40% of men.

Yohimbine (alpha-blocker)
This drug is not yet licensed.

○ (1998) *J Urol.* **159**: 433–6.
   A systematic review found this to be more effective than placebo. It has more side-effects than the other agents available.

National Strategy for Sexual Health and HIV (2001)

www.doh.gov.uk/nshs/index.htm
www.sxhealth.co.uk
Copies of the strategy can be obtained from the Department of Health, PO Box 777, London SE1 6LH.

In July 2001 a consultation document was published that outlined the Government's proposed strategy for sexual health and HIV. The main aim of the strategy is to prevent sexual causes of premature death and ill health, as well as to ensure that services are available for those patients who need them.

Local networks of providers will be based on three service levels.

Level 1: to be provided by GPs

- Sexual history and risk assessment
- Contraceptive information and services
- Pregnancy testing and referral
- Cervical cytology screening and referral
- Sexually transmitted disease (STD) testing for women
- Assessment and referral for men
- HIV testing and counselling
- Hepatitis B immunisation.

Level 2: intermediate care to be provided by primary care teams with a specialist interest, genito-urinary or family planning clinics

- IUD and contraceptive implants
- Testing and treatment of STDs
- Invasive STD testing for men
- Partner notification and contact tracing
- Vasectomy.

Level 3: specialist clinical teams across more than one primary care group

- Outreach contraceptive services
- Outreach for STD prevention
- Specialised infection management, including contact tracing
- Specialised HIV treatment and care.

A large proportion of GPs are already providing the majority of Level 1 services, the exceptions being HIV testing, counselling and contact tracing. The General Practitioners' Committee at present is not backing the strategy because of 'lack of resources, nurse time and training'. It is not thought that, with current workloads (implementing National Service Frameworks, etc.), GPs could take on the extra burden.

○ (2001) A Sexual Health and HIV Strategy for England. *BMJ*. **323**: 243–4.
This article gives a brief overview of some of the issues. Again the conclusion is that the £47.5 million to be invested between 2002 and 2004 is insufficient. If the target for reducing HIV and gonorrhoea by 25% by 2007 is met, it could save the Government £450 million. Further to this article, sexual abuse and assault services were not highlighted. The document was more concerned with 'disease prevention rather than health promotion'.

Paediatrics

Child health surveillance

In October 1999, the Royal College of General Practitioners published an information sheet of statistics and emphasised that the child health surveillance (CHS) programme is aimed at prevention of disease and illness at the earliest opportunity, as well as promoting good health and development.

In 1992, NHS regulations introduced payments for GPs who offered CHS for children under 5 years of age. To be eligible, the GP must be on the local CHS list.

There have been three editions of the Hall Report, *Health for all Children*.

- The first edition set out a programme of routine reviews for all preschool children.

- The second edition suggested how this might be delivered.

- The third edition was a response to evolving professional perceptions of preventative healthcare, coupled with rapid changes in the political context in which that care is provided.

The NSF for Children is being worked on following *The NHS Plan*.

Developmental dysplasia of the hip

This is a spectrum of conditions in which the head of the femur is partly or completely displaced from the acetabulum.

Risk factors include family history, breech presentation, oligohydramnios, postural deformities of the feet, being firstborn, Caesarean delivery, and female gender (sevenfold increase in risk).

The incidence is 1.25 in 100 births.

Early detection and conservative treatment are often successful and avoid the need for surgery. Routine screening (Ortalani and Barlow) (valid up to 3 months) misses up to 70% of cases. This is a falsely reassuring 'screening test' for both parents and doctors. Germany now has a universal ultrasound screening programme. The UK targets babies with risk factors or a positive Ortalani or Barlow, aiming for an ultrasound scan by 8 weeks.

Screening for hearing defects

- Around 840 children are born with permanent hearing impairment each year.

- Around 50% are not diagnosed until they are 18 months old.

- Around 25% are not diagnosed until they are 3 years old (i.e. the distraction test does not detect some cases early enough).

Permanent hearing impairment impacts on communication skills, educational attainment and quality of life. If there is intervention by 6 months, the outcome for all of the above, as well as the cost to society, is improved.

The Government has announced a new programme to screen all babies electronically within 48 hours of birth. This is called *otoacoustic emissions testing*. It has been known since the 1970s that for each sound heard by the ear, the ear produces a tiny corresponding sound ('echo') known as otoacoustic emission. This can now be measured by a computer and used clinically. Absence of an echo or a barely audible echo indicates that the child has a hearing problem. Sensitivity is in the range 80–90%, and costs would be less than those of the current distraction tests.

○ (2001) Prevalence of permanent childhood hearing impairment in the UK and implications for universal neonatal hearing screening: questionnaire-based ascertainment study. *BMJ.* **323**: 536–9.
This study highlights the importance of not becoming complacent, as not all cases of deafness are congenital. Progressive or late-onset problems (mainly genetic) account for 4–9% of all cases.

It is important to make parents aware that screening tests are just that – screening tests. If they have any worries or concerns, they need to seek advice from their GP or health visitor.

Sudden infant death syndrome (SIDS or 'cot death')

This is the unexpected and unexplained death of a child under 2 years of age.
    In 1994, the Back to Sleep Campaign was launched following the publication of a paper in 1990 which proved that sleeping prone increased the risk of cot death.
    Risk factors in the infant include the following:

- low birth weight
- prematurity
- sex (60% of cases are boys)
- multiple births
- high birth order (parity).

Risk factors in the parents include the following:

- young maternal age
- unmarried mothers
- maternal smoking in pregnancy
- *smoking after birth* – this increases the risk by fivefold, and is the biggest risk.

Environmental risk factors include the following:

- low socio-economic class
- sleeping prone
- winter

- overheating

- used cot mattresses.

  ○ (2002) *BMJ*. **325**: 1007–9.
    This study showed that used cot mattresses are a risk factor for SIDS.

  ○ (1999) Babies with parents: case-controlled study of factors influencing the risk of SIDS. *BMJ*. **319**: 1457–62.
    This study looked at 325 deaths (with 1300 controls). Sharing a bed was not a risk factor, but became one when it was associated with smoking, tiredness, alcohol consumption, overcrowding or thick duvets, especially if the infant was <14 weeks old.

It is estimated that 10–20% of SIDS cases involve child abuse. Covert video recording has increased awareness. However, it is fraught with potential problems, as was seen in the recently resolved Stoke case.

CONI (Care of the Next Infant) and the Foundation for the Study of Infant Deaths have been established to support parents. They provide counselling and apnoea alarms, among many other resources.

Vaccination programme

The immunisation schedule has saved more lives than any other public health measure, apart from the provision of clean water, and is now a victim of its own success.

The success of a vaccine is not the number of primary cases of the disease, but the number of secondary cases generated from the one primary source.

  ○ (2000) Two-dose MMR immunisation schedule: factors affecting maternal intention to vaccinate. *Br J Gen Pract*. **50**: 969–71.
    This study used a postal questionnaire which revealed the overwhelming finding that the diseases were no longer perceived to be important by parents/mothers, and the second vaccine was perceived to be unnecessary. The majority of mothers valued their GP's opinion.

  ○ (2003) MMR vaccine: how effective and how safe? *Drug Ther Bull*. **41**: 25–9.
    This article concludes that the weight of published evidence argues overwhelmingly in favour of MMR protection.

Is the MMR vaccination linked to autistic spectrum disorder?

The first signs of autism generally appear in the second year of life, which coincides with MMR vaccination. The incidence is unknown, as awareness and diagnostic criteria have changed in recent years. Autism has never been linked with the measles vaccine. However, the question arose with the introduction of mumps and rubella to produce a triple vaccine.

  ○ Wakefield *et al.* (1998) *Lancet*. **351**: 637–41.
    This study was published from the Royal Free Hospital in London. It described colitis with autism-like behaviour in 12 children. In eight of these children the parents remembered that the symptoms had started soon after the MMR vaccination. Team member Andrew Wakefield went on to state that the vaccine should be given as separate antigens at yearly intervals.
    It is worth noting that the study size is 12, whereas 13 million people have been vaccinated in the UK, and there have been 250 million vaccinations worldwide.

Wakefield and colleagues went on to review data that had been obtained prior to the introduction of MMR to the UK, and claimed that the evidence for its safety was very thin and granting of the product licence was premature.

○ (1998) MMR vaccination and autism 1998: déjà-vu pertussis and brain damage. *BMJ.* **316**: 715–16.

○ (1991) Is autism more common now than 10 years ago? *Br J Psychiatry.* **158**: 403–9.

○ (1999) Autism and the MMR vaccine: no epidemiological evidence for a causal association. *Lancet.*
The above studies showed that trends in autism were not related to the introduction of the MMR vaccine.

○ (2002) MMR vaccination and bowel problems or developmental regression in children with autism: population study. *BMJ.* **324**: 393–6.
This study looked at 278 children with autism (during the period 1979–1998), and found no link with the MMR vaccine.

A molecular pathology study (www.molpath.com) found that 83% of children with autism or bowel disorders were positive for measles virus in their intestines, compared with 7% of the controls. It was not established whether the children had had the MMR vaccination or whether this was due to infection.

○ (2001) MMR vaccine and the incidence of autism recorded by GPs: a time trend analysis. *BMJ.* **322**: 460–3.
This study shows that the increasing incidence of autism has continued over the last decade. If MMR was the cause, a plateau would have been expected, but this has not happened. The study provides evidence for the view that there is not a causal association between MMR and the risk of autism. It concludes that an explanation for the marked increase in the risk of diagnosis of autism during the past decade remains uncertain.

○ (2002) *Clin Evidence.* **7**: 331–40.
This dismissed the 1998 study that first claimed a link between autism and the MMR vaccine, pointing out that it was small, selective in its sample and lacked a control group. It concluded that there was no evidence that the MMR vaccine or the single measles vaccine was linked to autism.

Is the MMR linked to Crohn's disease?

1 Early exposure to measles does not appear to increase the risk of Crohn's disease. Two large studies from Denmark and the UK with appropriate controls showed no increased risk of Crohn's disease under these circumstances.

○ (1998) *BMJ.* **316**: 196–7.

2 The measles vaccine does not increase the risk of Crohn's disease.

○ (1995) *Lancet.* **345**: 1071–4.
A cohort of unmatched controls, differential dropout rates and different means of case ascertainment compared children from 1964 (immunised) with those from 1954 (not immunised) and suggested that there was an increased risk of Crohn's disease with vaccination.

○ (1997) *Lancet.* **350**: 764–6.
This study found no increased risk of Crohn's disease. This finding of no increased risk has been confirmed in Oxford and Finland.

As with all vaccines, there is ongoing national surveillance, and the Chief Medical Officer and the Committee on Safety of Medicines regularly review data.

The MMR scare in 1998 resulted in a 4% drop in uptake, reducing the immunisation rate to 85%. To eliminate measles, there needs to be an uptake of 94–96%.

MMR litigation

The High Court has said that 'no positive link has ever been established', and the Medical Research Council has confirmed this. Judges have gone on to say that 'unsubstantiated health scares endanger children and enrich lawyers'.

Single vaccines

Measles and mumps vaccine is unlicensed in the UK (rubella is licensed and available). If it is wanted, it must be obtained from abroad on a named-patient basis and it must be approved by the Medicines Control Agency.

Recently, Peter Mansfield from Lincolnshire has been referred to the General Medical Council for advice, as he has worked contrary to the public health department's advice and 'best medical opinion', by offering an alternative to MMR. Legally there is no case for professional misconduct.

Thiomersal in vaccines

Thiomersal is a mercury-based antimicrobial preservative that is found in some DTP preparations (and in some Hib vaccines outside the UK). Again this has caught media attention because of suspected links with autism.

It has never been part of live vaccines (MMR and BCG). The theoretical concerns are that in combination the cumulative mercury dose could exceed recommended safety levels.

The US and European regulatory bodies have recommended that thiomersal should be phased out. This has been endorsed by the World Health Organization, which has also stressed that if thiomersal-free vaccines are not available, vaccination programmes should not be compromised and children should still be vaccinated.

Note that three DTP vaccinations with or without Hib would give a maximum cumulative dose of 75 µg of ethylmercury – less than half of the 187 µg dose that is causing concern.

Autism

Autism is a lifelong developmental disability that affects social and communication skills with varying degrees of severity on a somatic–pragmatic scale. Onset is usually by the age of 3 years, but it can go undiagnosed. Early diagnosis enables behavioural therapy, facilitated communication and educational techniques to be introduced, hopefully improving the long-term outcome.

o (2000) Early identification of autism by the Checklist for Autism in Toddlers (CHAT). *J R Soc Med.* **93**: 521–5.
   This is a screening tool that can be used at the 18-month check by GPs or health visitors.

Checklist for Autism in Toddlers

Section A

1   Does your child enjoy being swung, bounced on your knee, etc.?   Yes/No
2   Does your child take an interest in other children?   Yes/No
3   Does your child like climbing on things (e.g. stairs)?   Yes/No
4   Does your child enjoy playing peek-a-boo/hide-and-seek?   Yes/No
5   **Does your child ever pretend, for example, to make a cup of tea using a toy cup and teapot, or pretend other things?**   **Yes/No**
6   Does your child ever use his/her index finger to point to *ask* for something?   Yes/No
7   **Does your child ever use his/her finger to point to indicate interest in something?**   **Yes/No**
8   Can your child play properly with small toys (e.g. bricks, cars) without just mouthing or fiddling with them?   Yes/No
9   Does your child ever bring objects over to show you something?   Yes/No

Section B

1   During the appointment, has the child made eye contact with you?   Yes/No
2   **Get the child's attention and then point across the room at an interesting object and say 'Oh look! There's a [name the toy]'. Does the child look across and see what you are pointing at?**   **Yes/No**
3   Get the child's attention and then give him/her a toy cup and teapot and say 'Can you make a cup of tea?' Does the child **pretend to make or drink the tea?**   **Yes/No**
4   **Say to the child 'Where is the light?'. Does the child point?**   **Yes/No**
5   Can the child build a tower of bricks? (how many?)   Yes/No

If the items in bold print are absent at 18 months, then the child is at high risk for a social communication disorder. If 'No' is the response to all five items, then the child is at high risk. If A7 and B4 are absent, then the child is at low risk for autism but should be rescreened about 1 month later.

Attention deficit hyperactivity disorder (ADHD)

Hyperactivity affects 1–2% of children. The consequences can be far-reaching, affecting education and causing behavioural problems and social isolation. Benefits can be obtained with medication, diet (there is anecdotal evidence for the benefits of excluding some food colourings and preservatives), behavioural therapy and educational support.

Access to treatment is influenced both by the parents and by the GP. Conflict, misunderstanding and dissatisfaction can occur if a parent's concerns are not taken seriously.

○ (1990) *Br J Gen Pract.* **49**: 563–71.
   This is a good overview that distinguishes between ICD-10 and DSM-IV classifications. The problems need to be present for at least 6 months and occur in two or more settings (i.e. not just at home). This disorder is defined by inattention, hyperactivity and impulsiveness.

○ (2003) *Br J Gen Pract.* **53**: 227–32.
   This discussion paper highlights diagnosis, aetiology, prognosis and the increasing role of primary care services in the recognition and treatment of ADHD. This role has not yet been defined.

Current research is focusing on cognitive processing, genetic factors, brain function abnormalities and the significance of comorbidity factors.

NICE guidelines for methylphenidate for ADHD, October 2000

- Methylphenidate is a sympathomimetic amine which works on dopamine receptors.

- It is used as part of the comprehensive treatment programme (paediatric and psychiatric).

- It is not licensed for use in children under 6 years, or in cases of thyrotoxicosis, tics, etc.

- Continued prescribing and monitoring may be performed by GPs under shared care.

NICE has called for further research to determine whether drug treatment, behavioural therapy or a combination of both is the best first-line treatment.

○ (1998) Attention deficit hyperactivity disorder. *Arch Dis Child.* **79**: 381–5.
   This comprehensive review of papers on ADHD highlights the need for specialist diagnosis and management. The role of the GP is 'strictly' one of support.

Ophthalmology

Macular degeneration

Age-related macular degeneration (AMD)

This is the most common cause of blind registration in industrialised countries. It impairs central vision and progresses slowly over a period of years.

Legal blindness is < 20/200 (6/60). This means that a person can see less than 20 feet (6 metres) when a normally-sighted person could see 200 feet (60 metres).

○ (2000) *BMJ.* **321**: 741–4.
   Clinical Evidence 2000 looked at a number of treatment options and these were reviewed in the above article. In four randomised controlled trials of thermal laser coagulation, benefits were seen with accurate, complete treatment, with high-quality angiography and experienced practitioners.

In photodynamic therapy with verteporfin dye, a non-thermal laser activates the dye once injected to close the new choroidal vessels (in exudative AMD). This treatment looks promising.

There is no real evidence for radiotherapy or submacular surgery in AMD.

○ (2001) Risk of macular degeneration in users of statins: cross-sectional study. *BMJ*. **323**: 375–6.
There were 379 patients in this trial, 7% of whom were using statins. It was found that 22% of non-statin users showed signs of macular degeneration, compared with 4% of statin users.

The authors of the above trial suggest three mechanisms that could link statin use with a lower risk of macular degeneration, although it should be noted that the confidence intervals were wide.

1 Statins may prevent the accumulation of basal linear deposits in Bruch's membrane which occurs with higher concentrations of cholesterol.

2 Antioxidant properties of statins might protect the outer retina from oxidative damage.

3 Simvastatin inhibits endothelial cell apoptosis and preserves ischaemic vasculature, perhaps maintaining a competent vascular supply to the macula.

○ (2003) Cholesterol-lowering drugs and risk of age-related maculopathy: prospective cohort study with cumulative exposure measurements. *BMJ*. **324**: 255–6.
This study from The Netherlands with 26 781 person-years follow-up found no association between cholesterol-lowering drugs and age-related maculopathy. The authors discussed the fact that previous studies had low statistical powers.

ENT

Sore throat

This is the most common, over-treated, controversial and mundane (or is it?) symptom in general practice.

The Cochrane Review looked at antibiotics and complications of sore throats, and concluded that antibiotics offered a small clinical benefit. They were found to reduce the risk of rheumatic fever by up to 30%, but this would be barely significant in the Western world. The incidence of acute otitis media was reduced by 25%.

If an antibiotic is necessary, which one? (MeReC Bulletin November 11, 1999)

A study of group A *Streptococcus* over the last 80 years has shown no development of resistance to penicillin.

○ (1998) *Pediatr Infect Dis J*. **17**: 377.

● Avoid ampicillin and amoxycillin, as if there is Epstein–Barr infection this will precipitate a maculopapular rash.

● Most clinical trials use penicillin V 250 mg four times a day for 10 days. This has been found to be more effective in eradicating group A *Streptococcus* than 5 or 7 days of treatment.

○ (1997) Randomised trial of prescribing strategies in managing sore throat. *BMJ*. **314**: 722–7.
This study looked at immediate prescription, no treatment or delayed prescribing in 716 patients. It found that 69% of people who were offered delayed prescribing did not use the script. The proportion of patients who were better by day 3 and the overall duration of illness did not differ between the groups.

○ (2000) Study comparing management of sore throats by GPs vs. nurses. *Br J Gen Pract*. **50**: 872–80.
In this study there was no random allocation, but rather the patients self-selected. Practice nurses were found to offer a safe and effective service for the treatment of sore throats in primary care in an emergency setting.

Acute otitis media

● Around 66% of cases are due to *Haemophilus influenzae* and *Streptococcus pneumoniae*.

● Around 25% are sterile.

● Around 10–20% are due to *Mycoplasma* and anaerobes.

● About 4% are viral (although titres are raised in 25%, possibly preceding bacterial infection).

Use of antibiotics

○ (2001) Pragmatic RCT of two prescribing strategies for childhood acute otitis media. *BMJ*. **322**: 336–42.
This randomised controlled trial in 351 children compared immediate treatment with antibiotics with a 72-hour wait-and-see policy. Those who were prescribed antibiotics showed a symptomatic benefit after 24 hours, had fewer disturbed nights and consumed slightly less paracetamol. There was no difference in school attendance, pain or distress. It was concluded that a wait-and-see approach was acceptable to most parents, and resulted in a 76% reduction in prescribing.

○ (2002) Predictors of poor outcome and benefits from antibiotics in children with acute otitis media: pragmatic randomised trial. *BMJ*. **325**: 22–5.
The aim of this trial was to identify children who were at higher risk of poor outcome (severity and length of illness). Predictors were earache lasting for more than 3 days, ear discharge, three or more previous courses of antibiotics (compared with none), higher temperature and vomiting. It was concluded that children without fever and vomiting were unlikely to benefit from antibiotics.

○ (2000) Primary care double-blind randomised trial of Amoxil vs. placebo in under-twos. *BMJ*. **320**: 350–4.
In this trial, 240 children (from 53 practices) were all given oxymetazoline 0.025% nosedrops. On day 4, 59% of the children on Amoxil still had earache, compared with 72% of those on placebo (NNT = 8). It was concluded that antibiotics were not of sufficient benefit, and that analgesia, watching and waiting were preferable.

Several meta-analyses have shown that the effectiveness of antibiotics is limited in terms of clinical improvement.

The advantages of antibiotics include the following:

● bacterial aetiology

● inexpensive and relatively safe

● reduction in complications (e.g. mastoiditis).

The disadvantages include the following:

- cost when prescribed in mass numbers
- possible loss of natural immunity
- may promote drug resistance
- may promote dependence on doctors' prescribing.

We need to ask whether we are justified in withholding antibiotics when we know that they do improve symptoms in children, especially in those who are too young to express their symptoms, especially of pain.

Glue ear

This is the most common cause of conductive hearing loss in children aged 2–5 years. Hearing loss has knock-on effects on speech development, school performance in writing and spelling, and behaviour (may be either over-boisterous or clingy).

Around 50% of cases resolve spontaneously within 3 months.

○ (1998) *Thorax*. **53**: 50–6.
This meta-analysis showed that causes include parental smoking.
   Grommets are an important and controversial issue in terms of resource implications. Repeat insertion is necessary in up to 30% of children.

○ (2001) TARGET (Trial of Alternative Regimens for Glue Ear) study. *Clin Otolaryngol*. **26**: 417–24.

○ UK Medical Research Council trial
These trials showed that grommet insertion resulted in significant improvement in quality of life as well as hearing in children aged 3–6 years. Problems included long-term hearing loss, persistent perforation and otorrhoea. The trials also confirmed the long-term benefit of adenoidectomy.

○ (2001) Behaviour and developmental effects of otitis media with effusion into the teens. *Arch Dis Child*. **85**: 91–5.
This longitudinal study of 1000 children during the period 1972–73 in New Zealand found that otitis media with effusion was associated with behavioural problems, especially inattentive behaviour well into the teens. It had a statistically significant effect on lowering of IQ, especially verbal IQ.

Gastric reflux in children can involve the reflux of gastric juices via the Eustachian tube into the middle ear. This can cause inflammation and ideal conditions for secondary infection.

○ (2001) Otitis externa in UK general practice: a survey using a general practice research database. *Br J Gen Pract*. **51**: 533–8.
The 1997 database revealed the following trends. An excess of cases was seen towards the end of summer (possibly reflecting swimming-related infections). Patients with eczema did not show greater persistence of otitis media, but they did have a higher rate of recurrence. Disease persistence was reduced by the use of eardrops containing steroids with or without antibiotic. However, this was not the case with oral antibiotic (neither treatment reduced recurrence rates).

Back pain

- Around 60–80% of the population will experience back pain at some time in their life.

- Up to 90% of acute episodes resolve within 6 weeks.

- Around 7% of people consult their GP each year with back pain.

- A total of 120 million working days per year are lost as a result of back pain.

Management

○ (1999) *BMJ*. **319**: 279–83.
This study showed that early access to a doctor (3 days) and a physiotherapist (1 week) for exercise for new-onset back pain was associated with a good outcome.

○ (1997) *Br J Gen Pract*. **47**: 647–52.
This systematic review of bed rest recommended that patients with acute lower back pain should remain active.

○ (1999) *BMJ*. **318**: 1662–7.
This study showed that premorbid state is a good clinical indicator of patients who will go on to develop chronic lower back pain.

Early mobilisation increases speed of recovery, decreases length of time off work and decreases the number of recurrences.

The Royal College of General Practitioners has published guidelines for lower back pain on their website, emphasising red flags to look out for and management options.
www.rcgp.org.uk

Red flags are symptoms and conditions that require urgent imaging, blood tests and referral. They include the following:

- premorbid history of carcinoma, TB, drug abuse or HIV (cause of immunosuppression and infection)

- drugs (e.g. steroids)

- symptoms of night sweats, fever, loss of weight

- new structural deformity (e.g. kyphosis)

- widespread neurology:
  - cauda equina symptoms (*need immediate referral* as there is a risk of permanent damage and incontinence)
    (i)   loss of sphincter control
    (ii) bilateral neurological leg pain
    (iii) saddle loss of sensation.

Osteoarthritis

Around 20–25% of visits to GPs relate to the musculoskeletal system. Most of these cases involve osteoarthritis.

Osteoarthritis, by definition, cannot be cured. Local corticosteroid injections are worth trying.

Management

o   (2000) *BMJ.* **321**: 936–40.
    This is a useful review of the medical management of osteoarthritis.

Diet

Other than weight loss, specific diets have no role to play in the management of rheumatic conditions. However, there are reports of vitamin C reducing rates of progression.

Exercise

Exercise improves muscular tone and joint function, so should not be avoided.

o   (2002) Home-based exercise programme for knee pain and knee osteoarthritis: randomised controlled trial. *BMJ.* **325**: 752–5.
    This trial found that simple home exercises can significantly reduce knee pain over a 2-year period.

Glucosamines

These are available as a dietary supplement, which is expensive.

Glucosamine sulphate is a natural substance that forms proteoglycans (part of the articular cartilage). It is thought to be chondroprotective.

o   (2002) *Drug Ther Bull.* **40**: 81–3.
    This suggests that doses of 1500 mg/day probably give modest symptom relief, similar to that obtained with NSAIDs.

o   Cochrane Review, 2001
    In 13 trials in which glucosamine was compared with placebo, glucosamine was found to be superior in all but one trial.

o   (2001) *BMJ.* **322**: 673.
    This randomised controlled trial showed improved symptoms compared to placebo. There have been similar trials for chondroitin, which is also chondroprotective.

o   (2001) *BMJ.* **322**: 1439–40.
    This editorial provides an interesting overview.

Intra-articular hyaluronic acid gives symptomatic benefit and has a longer duration of action than triamcinolone. This has been confirmed in randomised controlled trials.

COX-2 inhibitors

- Around 15% of people on long-term NSAIDs develop ulcers, accounting for 2000 deaths per year.

- In 1999, more than £170 million was spent on NSAIDs, not including the co-prescribing of gastroprotective agents.

- COX-2 inhibitors are as effective as other NSAIDs in reducing inflammation and pain.

There have been 53 randomised controlled trials (involving 61 731 patients) looking at rofecoxib, celecoxib, meloxicam and etodolac. These drugs are more effective than placebo in reducing pain and improving function. Their gastrointestinal side-effect profile is better than that of NSAIDs. The cardiovascular and renal side-effects are as yet unresolved.

○ (2002) Efficacy and safety of COX-2 inhibitors. *BMJ*. **325**: 607–8.
This editorial gives a good overview of recent trials, including CLASS (which found a lower incidence of symptomatic ulcers compared with ibuprofen and diclofenac) and VIGOR.

○ (2002) Efficacy, tolerability and upper gastrointestinal safety of celecoxib for treatment of osteoarthritis and rheumatoid arthritis: systematic review of randomised controlled trials. *BMJ*. **325**: 619–23.
This review found celecoxib to be as effective as other NSAIDs. Celecoxib also had improved tolerability and gastrointestinal safety.

NICE guidelines on cyclo-oxygenase inhibitors

- These drugs are indicated for pain and stiffness in inflammatory arthritis and short-term pain relief in osteoarthritis.

- They are not recommended for routine use.

- They are recommended for those over 65 years of age who are taking other drugs that could cause gastrointestinal side-effects (e.g. steroids and anticoagulants), and those patients who have existing gastrointestinal problems.

These recommendations were challenged by the drug manufacturers for not allowing wider prescribing. This delayed publication of the guidelines.

Osteoporosis

This is defined as 'a skeletal disorder characterised by low bone mass and micro-architectural deterioration of bone tissue with a consequent increase in bone fragility and susceptibility to fracture' (NHS Consensus Development Conference).

○ (1993) *Ann Intern Med*. **94**: 646–50.

The WHO definition is as follows:

- Osteoporosis: bone density >2.5 SD below the mean.

- Osteopenia: bone density >1 SD below the mean.

Note that one definition is a pathological process and the other is an arbitrary point on a scale. The T-score criteria were proposed for epidemiological studies to compare populations and for defining thresholds in clinical trials. They were not intended for diagnosis or management decisions in individual cases.

- Osteoporosis causes >200 000 fractures per year (mainly wrist, vertebral and hip fractures).

- It costs the Government £1.5 billion per year (87% of this is due to hip fractures).

- A third of women and a sixth of men will have one or more osteoporotic fractures.

- One in five hip fracture patients die within 1 year, 50% have severely impaired mobility, and a third of vertebral fractures cause chronic pain (i.e. there is a huge impact on morbidity and mortality).

Risk factors

These include the following:

- postmenopausal women

- early menopause (before 45 years of age)

- immobility

- long-term steroid use (recent Royal College of Physicians guidelines)

- previous fragility fracture

- high systolic blood pressure (higher rate of bone loss)

- secondary causes
  - alcoholism
  - thyroid problem (hypothyroidism and hyperthyroidism)
  - liver disease
  - malabsorption
  - hypogonadism in men.

Around 50% of men and 10% of women will have a secondary cause.
   Genetic factors are not thought to be a big issue.

○ (1999) Genetic factors and osteoporotic fractures in elderly people: prospective 25-year follow-up. *BMJ.* **319**: 1334–7.

Treatment

Prevention/life style changes

- Stop smoking; avoid excess alcohol; take regular weight-bearing exercise.
- Fall prevention – safety at home.
- Protection of sites of high impact. Hip protectors are of proven benefit.

  ○ (1996) *Effect Health Care Bull.* **2**: 1–16.
  This study showed a reduction in fractures of up to 50% as a result of the use of hip protectors in nursing homes.

Calcium supplements

- The recommended daily dose of 700 mg for those over 50 years of age is thought to be too low (1 g is suggested).
- This is no evidence that calcium reduces fractures unless it is taken with vitamin D.

Vitamin D

- The recommended daily dose of 400 iU is too low for fracture prevention; 800 iU is recommended.
- Two trials have shown that vitamin D and calcium reduced the risk of fracture by up to 50% over 5 years.
- There are problems with regard to which vitamin D preparation to use. Trials are still under way.

Bisphosphonates

  ○ (2001) *Drug Ther Bull.* **39**: 68–72.
  Aledronate decreases hip fractures by 50% in postmenopausal women.

  ○ (1996) *Lancet.* **348**: 1535–41.
  Etidronate has been licensed for prevention of bone loss in postmenopausal women in 90-day cycles. There is no evidence to suggest that it reduces fractures. Risedronate reduces vertebral fractures post-menopausally. However, it is not clear how long these drugs should be used for.

Hormone replacement therapy

A meta-analysis suggests that this yields a relative risk reduction of 40% for fractures. However, the benefits are lost within 5 years of stopping HRT.

Tibolone (bleed-free preparation of HRT)

This increases bone mass density in the spine over a period of 2 years.

Selective oestrogen-receptor modulators (SERMs) (e.g. raloxifene)

These decrease the fracture rate by 30% over 3 years, as shown by randomised controlled trials.

Screening

Fractures occur late in life and there are no symptoms prior to this. All women over 65 years of age in the USA are screened. However, there is no universal policy in the UK.

Royal College of Physicians guidelines, 1999

These guidelines suggest that DEXA scanning should be offered to individuals with risk factors, as well as to those with a low bone mass density (<19) and those with a strong family history (despite the Finnish study which concluded that genetic factors were not important).

Population screening is not offered at present, as there are still problems to be resolved regarding its management.

DEXA (dual X-ray absorptiometry)

○   (1996) *BMJ*.
     This meta-analysis showed that DEXA is currently the best method of assessment.

Assessment of severity may aid management decisions.

Remember that low bone mass density on DEXA is only one risk factor for fractures. Several studies have shown that wrist or heel ultrasound scans may be as effective as DEXA scanning in predicting fracture risk.

○   (2001) For and against: bone densitometry is not a good predictor of hip fracture. *BMJ*. **323**: 795–9.
     This article concluded that bone densitometry is not a good predictor of hip fractures. This is a sensibly written piece which advocates looking at age and secondary risk factors as predictors of hip fracture.

Useful information can be obtained from the National Osteoporosis Society (www.nos.org.uk)

Alcohol misuse

Around 5% of the population are alcohol dependent. As GPs, we are aware that this accounts for around a third of our patients. A much higher proportion misuses alcohol.

In men, alcohol consumption of >300 g/week is associated with increased blood pressure and risk of stroke. Drinking 1–4 units/day in men and 1–2 units/day in women on 5 to 6 days of the week appears to be protective against coronary heart disease and possibly stroke.

Tackling those patients who misuse alcohol and getting them to recognise that they are drinking too much is probably the area where we as GPs have the biggest impact.

There is no official policy or strategy for alcohol dependence, but if or when it is produced it will need to consider various issues, including licensing hours, alcohol availability, cost and drink driving, as well as health services and resources.

Brief intervention by a GP can be effective, depending on where the patient is in the cycle of change.

○ (1988) Randomised controlled trial of GP intervention in patients with excessive alcohol consumption. *BMJ.* **297**: 663–8.
   If detox is going to be necessary, you need to assess the general health of your patient. If they are malnourished, inpatient detox may be a safer option.

The Chief Medical Officer's Update 35 (January 2003) highlighted the fact that 40 000 people per year die from alcohol-related causes, and there is currently a National Harm Reduction Strategy consultation in progress.
www.doh.gov.uk/alcoholstrategy.htm

Screening tools

○ (2003) Screening in brief intervention trials targeting excessive drinkers in general practice: systematic review and meta-analysis. *BMJ.* **327**: 536–40.
   Even brief advice can reduce excessive drinking but the use of screening in general practice is still unclear.

CAGE questionnaire

• Have you ever felt you should **C**ut down on your drinking?

• Have you ever been **A**nnoyed by someone criticising your drinking?

• Have you ever felt **G**uilty about your drinking?

• Have you ever had an **E**ye-opener (early-morning drink) to steady your nerves/ get rid of your hangover?

A score of ⩾2 has a high correlation with alcoholism, but this screening tool has a low sensitivity and specificity.

○ (2001) Screening properties of questionnaires. *Br J Gen Pract.* **51**: 206–17.

AUDIT (Alcohol Use Disorder Identification Test)

This WHO screening tool is thought to be a more suitable screening test for excessive drinking at the less severe end of the spectrum. It has been found to have a higher sensitivity and specificity than the CAGE questionnaire.

o (1993) *Addiction.* **88**: 791–803.

o (2002) Screening and brief intervention for excessive alcohol use: qualitative interview study of the experiences of GPs. *BMJ.* **325**: 870–2.
This study showed that once patients had been identified by screening, doctors found it difficult to establish a rapport and ensure compliance with intervention. The programme needed considerable resources, and it was concluded that screening created more problems than it solved for the participating doctors.

o (2000) Managing the heavy drinker in primary care. *Drug Ther Bull.* **38**: 60–4.
This article gives a good overview on diagnosis, screening tools and management, including withdrawal and vitamin supplementation. It highlights the importance of screening in the primary health-care team.

o (2001) Alcohol consumption and the risk of dementia: the Rotterdam study. *BMJ.* **359**: 281–6.
This prospective population-based study of 7983 people aged over 55 years found that people who consumed up to three glasses of alcohol per day had a significantly lower risk of developing vascular dementia.

Drug misuse

It is estimated that 250 000 people in the UK have problems related to drug misuse.

This is a growing area of concern in that all GPs will encounter patients who misuse drugs. It is our responsibility to ensure that we provide care for general health needs as well as drug-related problems, referring patients to specialist services where appropriate.

The Home Office collects data on drug misuse, and this shows that increasing numbers of people are misusing drugs. GPs no longer have to supply the names of addicts.

Modernising the Health Service looks at drug issues in part, and aims to provide targeted prevention activity for at least 30% of those young people who are most vulnerable to drug misuse.

Guidelines on Clinical Management was first published in 1984 and is regularly updated (most recently in 1999).

Although addicts want GPs to be involved in their treatment, doctors should not be pressurised into accepting responsibilities beyond their level of expertise. This issue has recently been brought to our attention again in a case where a GP was charged with manslaughter when one of his teenage patients died of a methadone overdose. This highlights the importance of good support being provided from secondary care in a shared-care approach. An initial thorough and accurate assessment is mandatory.

In March 2001 the Department of Health issued a statement on the use of buprenorphine in the treatment of drug addiction. It has been recognised for use in opiate withdrawal, detoxification and maintenance, and in randomised controlled trials it has shown comparable success to methadone.

Obesity

Obesity is defined as a BMI >30 kg/m^2.

It is a growing medical, public health and economic problem. The main increase in mortality is related to cardiovascular disease.

o (2002) *JAMA*. **287**: 356–9.
   This study looks at genetic reasons for obesity in patients with a 'metabolic syndrome' (i.e. waist circumference >102 cm in men, or >88 cm in women, increased triglyceride and fasting blood glucose levels, and reduced HDL-cholesterol levels).

Tackling Obesity in England was published by the National Audit Office in February 2001. It inspiringly said that we needed national guidelines for primary care.

Two articles have recently looked at intervention in primary schools to reduce risk factors for obesity.

o (2001) Active Programmes Promoting Lifestyle Education in Schools (APPLES). *BMJ*. **323**: 1027–9.
   This article evaluated the implementation and effect of primary school intervention to reduce risk factors for obesity. The intervention consisted of a multidisciplinary, multi-agency health promotion programme which produced changes at school level. The long-lasting effects need to be monitored into adulthood.

o (2001) Randomised controlled trial of primary school-based intervention to reduce risk factors for obesity. *BMJ*. **323**: 1029–32.
   The intervention here consisted of teacher training, modification of school meals, physical education, etc. The trial concluded that there was little effect on children's behaviour other than a modest increase in vegetable consumption.

o (2002) Population strategies to prevent obesity. *BMJ*. **325**: 728–9.
   In order to prevent obesity, a series of population-based strategies have been proposed. The emphasis is on changing the environment. In this editorial, Professor David Crawford raises some interesting points.

Orlistat (Xenical)

This pancreatic lipase inhibitor can block up to 30% of fat absorption (causing steatorrhoea, wind, etc.). NICE has published guidelines on its use. Criteria include BMI $>$ 30 kg/m^2 (>28 kg/m^2 if associated with risk factors). Prior to starting, the patient needs to have lost 2.5 kg over 4 weeks, and once started, they need to lose 5% of their body weight over 12 weeks, or else discontinue treatment. This drug can be used for a maximum of 2 years.

Sibutramine (Reductil)

NICE have published guidelines with the same indications for prescription as for orlistat.

Exercise

Active adults live longer!

Obesity in the UK, in both children and adults, is increasing. This has numerous implications for health (e.g. non-insulin-dependent diabetes mellitus, coronary heart disease, osteoarthritis, etc). Exercise is effective for long-term weight reduction/regulation. The gold standard randomised controlled trials are difficult in terms of blinding. Below is a summary of what are known to date to be the beneficial effects of exercise.

Effects on cardiovascular disease

- Exercise reduces primary and secondary cardiovascular disease.
- Coronary heart disease reduced by 20–30% in men.
- Stroke could be reduced by 30–40%.
- Blood pressure can be reduced by up to 10 mmHg systolic and 8 mmHg diastolic.
- Exercise increases HDL-cholesterol levels.

Musculoskeletal effects

- Exercise has been shown to increase mobility and reduce falls in the elderly.
- It can reduce the rate of hip fracture by up to 50%.
- Weight-bearing exercise increases bone density.

Psychiatric effects

- Exercise reduces and relieves anxiety.
- It appears to have an antidepressant effect.

Other effects

- Exercise can prevent non-insulin-dependent diabetes mellitus (NIDDM) in 25% of cases.
- It improves glucose tolerance in NIDDM.
- People who exercise live longer.
- Graded aerobic exercise improves fatigue, functional capacity and fitness in patients with chronic fatigue syndrome.

The role of the GP and primary care is unclear in that although we are ideally placed, we lack a strong consensus on how to approach this, and which exercise programmes would benefit which patients.

The health authority advice is to take 30–40 minutes of moderate exercise five to seven times a week, although shorter bouts of more physical exercise can give similar benefits.

'Exercise on prescription' is something to be wary of, as the word 'prescription' implies a full understanding of the possible side-effects and complications. The defence unions have advised against prescribing exercise if you do not have the skill to evaluate the patient. However, you can recommend it.

Part 2

Introduction

Part 2 is dedicated to the latest policies and the more ambiguous topics. From a general practice point of view this will eventually inevitably form part of your working knowledge. In exam terms, although you need to have an understanding of such issues, you are most likely to get oral questions in the MRCGP exam relating to this book. If you are a quick writer you will be able to get some points down in the written exam.

As with Part 1, flick through the different sections to get a handle on what is included and where it features.

A brief history of general practice

The first reference to general practice was around 200 years ago, and since then development has been slow but has created an essentially stable primary healthcare system.

1815	Recognised profession
1841	Royal Pharmaceutical Society of Great Britain established
1858	General Medical Council established to control standards and conduct, educate doctors, and protect public and profession from quacks
1911	David Lloyd George set up medical insurance
1920	Dawson Report on the future of primary and secondary care
1942	Beveridge Report on the setting up of a Welfare State
1946	NHS set up under Labour Government
1952	College of General Practitioners founded (Royal status granted in 1967)
1966	General Practice Charter – main principles: better pay, seniority, group practices, designated area allowances, financial recognition of out-of-hours and reimbursement schemes for staff salaries
1968	Recommendation of three-year vocational training scheme by Royal College of General Practitioners on medical education; compulsory from 1982
1971	Direct access to laboratory facilities
1990	Government paper *Working for Patients* published

- Set performance targets
- Increased percentage income from patient numbers
- New item-of-service payments to encourage minor surgery, child health surveillance, health promotion and deprived-area incentives

1991	Fundholding commenced
1995	General Medical Council's *Good Medical Practice*
1996	White Paper on *Primary Care: Delivering the Future*
1997	Summative assessment
1998	Primary care groups developed to replace fundholding
2000	NHS Plan
2002	New World Organization of Family Doctors (WONCA) definition of general practice

The future of general practice

Parliament is responsible for the entire NHS. General practice is here to provide a primary care service to the whole population (i.e. it is the first point of contact with the NHS, together with Accident and Emergency, Family Planning, NHS Direct, genito-urinary clinics, etc.). Everyone in the UK has the right of access to a GP.

Our role is demand led and covers preventative healthcare, acute and chronic diseases, business, research, audit, training and teaching, as well as co-ordination between services for patients and their families.

Over the past 50 years there have been four major changes:

1 in 1948, the NHS was established

2 in 1966, the GP Charter was introduced

3 in 1990, the new contract was introduced

4 in 2000, the NHS Plan was published.

As part of the ongoing development, the discussion document *Shaping Tomorrow: Issues Facing General Practice in the New Millennium* was issued by Chris Mihill of the General Practitioners' Committee (GPC) of the BMA. It has collected views from the profession, politicians and patients, addressing topics such as what patients want and what model should replace the 'Dr Finlay icon of the all-purpose, 24-hour, home-visiting family doctor'. There are 12 chapters in the document, from which we have selected and summarised what we consider to be the most important issues.

My doctor or any doctor?

The drive to make speedy access a primary care priority is not necessarily the main concern of patients. Two main patient groups have emerged, namely the essentially well who value easy access to healthcare with staff who are able to deal with their problems, and those with chronic diseases who prefer to see their own doctor.

Many GPs regard the personal relationship with patients as central to what they do, while others view it as a fading asset due to modern-day careers. In many busy urban practices the concept of 'my doctor' is already meaningless, and some feel that the future will be about 'one-hit' consultations.

Interestingly, in countries where there is little continuity of care (or records) there are higher rates of investigation. Here lies an obvious argument for continuity of both care and records.

Should GPs let go and use the primary healthcare team?

This question really focuses on the purpose of the consultation, and although most patients are happy to see a nurse for triage or treatment of a minor illness, there is the flip side of the coin that no consultation is trivial, but rather it is an opportunity for discovering hidden agendas and health promotion. If such points of contact were lost, would the 'holistic care' approach be jeopardised? Would patients view nurse appointments as second-class?

Interestingly, although over the last 10 years in the USA nurse care has been dramatically increased, there has not been a reduced demand on doctors. Is this because demand is being fuelled? Or is it because doctors are good at dealing opportunistically with problems when the reason for attendance is otherwise trivial? Either way, further cost analyses are needed to determine the overall economic implications of nurse practitioners and whether they really do reduce doctors' workload.

Independent contractor status vs. salaried service

Independent contractor status is deemed to allow GPs greater control over their working practice, hours and staff, and to enable them to act as advocates on behalf of their patients. This is thought to encourage innovation, change and efficiency. This style of contract means that the Government gets more for its money. If GPs were all salaried for certain hours (i.e. 40 hours per week), there would be more doctors needed and consequently more would be spent on wages.

However, there is a widely held belief that independence is an illusion and will become increasingly so in the world of primary care trusts, clinical governance, National Service Frameworks and the Commission for Health Improvement (CHI). Taking a salaried stance does not mean that you lose your autonomy, or that you can no longer be an advocate for your patient.

The question arises as to whether it is possible to be an independent practitioner without being an independent contractor.

A job for life or a portfolio career?

Women, ethnic doctors and non-principals are an under-used resource. Young doctors are wanting flexible careers, to work part-time, the chance to move between practices or even to mix general practice with other careers. This situation needs to be recognised and addressed in order to help keep morale high within the profession and stop doctors leaving. Personal Medical Services (PMS) pilots are exploring these options and are supported nationally (stating the obvious, as this is where the funding is coming from).

Gatekeeper: is there still a role? Will walk-in centres and NHS Direct change the game?

Walk-in centres and NHS Direct have increased the number of access points to primary care. It is anticipated that in the future this or another form of triage will be used in the first instance, with GPs further down the line.

Is this a way of tackling the social aspect of modern-day medicine for disbanded families (the grandmother role)? Will GPs be expected to take on specialist roles because they are a cheaper option than secondary care?

GP supporters recognise that we protect patients from unnecessary over-investigation, so by definition are cost-saving.

Clinical autonomy: does it have a place any more?

This in a way goes back to the independent contractor status issue in that, whatever your opinion, we live in the world of NICE, National Service Frameworks, guidelines, protocols, evidence-based medicine, CHI and clinical governance.

Does autonomy mean anything any more? The answer is yes, it does. There has to be autonomy. Although there are guidelines, you do not have to follow them if your patient dictates otherwise. The time when this will become problematic is when pay or PMS contracts are performance related (audit, etc.). It would have to include these scenarios to account for shortfalls in audit numbers, if this was an issue.

Primary care groups: working together or professional straitjacket?

Primary care groups/primary care trusts mean increasing accountability and increasing pressure to deliver consistent care in an evidence-based way. This is not an easy task – are we compromising our patients by becoming the body for distributing services with an 'essentially inadequate budget'?

Promoting quality: what makes a good GP? Will revalidation stop bad doctors?

This chapter looks at issues such as quality (which in itself will not mean the same to all of us), consistency and increasing the number of GP specialists (i.e. additional GP roles contracted by the primary care trust – patients would then be referred to secondary care from that point).

Future pressures

This looks at what patients want (not necessarily what they need), funding and rationing. Pressure will come from all areas – the elderly, genetics, the Internet, consumerism and patient expectations – all of which will drive standards.

Clare Raynor of the Patients' Association believes that the way forward lies in seeing that patients are as much a part of the healthcare team as the professionals.

Internationally, general practice in the UK is often regarded as a model of primary care. It is important that it remains so.

Shaping Tomorrow concludes that change is being imposed by the Government (like it or not!) and the challenge is to retain those parts of general practice which are valued by, and bring satisfaction to, patients and doctors. To do this, we need to define what is special and central to what we do, and then fight to keep it. It is better to try and shape tomorrow rather than have it imposed on us.

As yet it is not clear what the 'Millennium GP' should look like! (Yes, it actually says that!)

○ (2001) Personal care from GPs. *Br J Gen Pract.*
   This Oxfordshire study found that patients valued the doctor–patient relationship more highly than prompt access, especially if the patient had psychological or significant health problems.

NHS Plan

This is a 10-year reform plan/vision for the NHS that was published in July 2000. Although it continues to underpin the founding principles of the NHS ('access to care for all on the basis of need, not ability to pay') it will bring about far-reaching changes across the NHS.

There are five main challenges that need to be addressed:

1 *partnership* – across the NHS to ensure the best possible care

2 *performance* – setting and delivering high standards within the NHS

3 *professions* – the wider NHS workforce must work together to deliver services for patients, breaking down traditional barriers

4 *patient care* – delivery should be fast and convenient, listening to need and letting patients know their rights

5 *prevention* – promoting healthy living across all societies, and tackling variations in care.

In January 2001, the Department of Health published *Primary Care, General Practice and the NHS Plan*, which covered much the same ground, but was aimed more specifically at primary-care professionals. We have broken these down into digestible chunks with the initial time-scale plans.

Planned investment

Chronic underfunding has been acknowledged, and there is now a plan for sustained increases in funding.

By 2004:

- 6500 more therapists
- 2000 more GPs
- 7500 more consultants
- 20 000 more nurses
- 1000 more medical student places
- 7000 extra beds in hospital/intermediate care.

By 2010:

- 100+ new hospitals
- 500 one-stop primary care centres

- 3000+ GP premises will be modernised.

In addition, childcare support will be available for NHS staff, with 100 on-site nurseries.

Information technology/accessibility

By 2002:

- all GPs will have access to the NHS net.

By 2004:

- access to electronic personal medical patient records (EPRs); 75% of hospitals and 50% of primary care trusts and primary healthcare teams will have implemented EPRs
- electronic prescribing of medication
- a single call to NHS Direct will be a one-stop gateway to out-of-hours care.

By 2005:

- electronic booking of appointments
- local health services to have provision for telemedicine
- maximum wait no longer than 48 hours for routine GP appointment, or 24 hours to see a practice nurse
- maximum wait for any stage of treatment no longer than 6 months (3 months by 2008).

General practice

By 2001:

- every primary care group must have in place a system to monitor practice referral rates.

By 2002:

- a third of all GPs will be expected to be working to PMS contracts.

By 2003:

- primary care groups will have become primary care trusts
- occupational health services will be extended to GPs and their staff.

By 2004:

- there will be extended nurse prescribing (over 50% will be able to prescribe).

New contracts are expected for single-handed practices unless the Red Book can be renegotiated.
There will be stronger partnerships with the pharmaceutical industry.
PMS contracts will expand.

Patient involvement

By 2002:

- patient advocates in every trust
- PALS (Patient Advocacy and Liaison Service).

There will also be:

- further overhaul of the complaints system; the NHS will act on concerns before they become complaints
- increased lay input at every level, including advising NICE
- patient views on local health services to help decide how much cash they receive
- letters about patient care copied to the patient
- if an operation is cancelled, the patient can choose the date within 28 days or the hospital will pay for the operation to be performed at another hospital of the patient's choosing.

Other points raised

These include the following:

- anti-ageism policy
- nursing care in nursing homes to be free
- better access to dental care
- better diet, with fruit available in schools for 4- to 6-year-olds
- retirement health checks
- modern contracts for doctors
- new care trusts to commission health and social care in a single organisation.

Out-of-hours care/24-hour responsibility

Patient demand for out-of-hours care has been steadily increasing over the last 40 years. This is reflected by the increase in night visits claimed and the attendance in casualty departments. Deputising services and out-of-hours co-operatives have changed the way in which GPs fulfil their 24-hour responsibility to their patients.

Raising Standards for Patients: New Partnerships in Out-of-Hours Care was published in October 2000. It made various recommendations, including:

- triage through a single call to NHS Direct by 2004 (for all out-of-hours care)

- electronic records which out-of-hours staff can access

- quality assessments of medical staff, organisations and access through clinical governance.

The report would allow us as GPs to end 24-hour responsibility. However, if the organisation covering out-of-hours care failed to meet certain standards, the primary care group/trust could return the responsibility to the GP.

○ (2001) *Br J Gen Pract*. **51**: 719–23.
This qualitative study of 30 patients aged 65–85 years showed that elderly patients preferred out-of-hours care provided by someone who knew their medical history. They were distrustful of nurse advice.

NHS Direct

NHS Direct is a 24-hour telephone advice line staffed by 'specially trained' nurses that aims to empower patients by giving them 'easier and faster information about health, illness and the NHS' (i.e. by going some way towards the Government's vision of a modernised healthcare system).

At present it is mainly being used by patients for reassurance and as an out-of-hours service (72% of calls were made after GP surgeries had closed), and caller satisfaction rates are reported to be high (*Evaluation of NHS Direct First-Wave Sites: First Interim Report to the Department of Health*). This report also highlighted the fact that different advice was being offered by different centres for identical 'dummy cases' in the pilot stages of NHS Direct.

Positive points include the following:

- aimed at reducing NHS workload

- easy access

- empowers patients

- encourages self-care

- accompanying NHS Direct healthcare guide.

Concerns include the following:

- may fuel workload/demand

- issues surrounding continuity of care

- missed diagnosis with telephone consultations

- will there be adequate integration with out-of-hours cover; if not, this may cause confusion

- not equally accessible to all (e.g. deaf, elderly, mentally ill, non-English-speaking).

The NHS Direct healthcare guide was written by Dr Ian Banks (a GP in Northern Ireland) with the help of an editorial board. The literature is designed to be used in conjunction with NHS Direct. It gives basic information, using narratives and flow charts on health and illness, as well as giving a guide as to when patients should contact NHS Direct for further advice. It is available both as a printed booklet and on the Internet (www.nhsdirect.nhs.uk). Again a major problem is promotion and accessibility to those most in need (e.g. the socially deprived or illiterate).

NHS Direct is part of the NHS and has been designed to work alongside other services, its current role being to provide instant access to a qualified nurse. The next main goal is that it will triage all out-of-hours calls by 2004 (as set out briefly in the NHS Plan). It further expanded following an independent review, *Raising Standards for Patients. New Partnerships in Out-of-Hours Care*, published in October 2000.

To date, NHS Direct has not reduced pressure on the NHS, nor has it appeared to uncover extra demand that was previously unrecognised.

○ (2000) Impact of NHS Direct on demand for immediate care: observational study. *BMJ*. **321**: 150–3.

The National Audit Office's report *NHS Direct in England* found:

- some co-operatives (in the North East) experienced an 18% reduction in calls when callers were transferred to NHS Direct first

- high levels of customer satisfaction.

○ (2002) NHS Direct audited. *BMJ*. **324**: 558–9.
This is a quirky editorial on the set-up and financing of NHS Direct – worth a read.

A further analysis in Derbyshire in August 2001 showed that GP workload was eased by 34%.

○ (2002) Impact of NHS Direct on general practice consultations during the winter 1999–2000: analysis of routinely collected data. *BMJ*. **325**:1397–8.
The introduction of NHS Direct had no impact on the number of consultations for influenza-like illness and other respiratory infections. NHS Direct was not introduced to increase or decrease the number of consultations, but rather to make them more appropriate. This issue was not looked at in the study.

Walk-in centres

These have been developed to cover part of the demand for out-of-hours care, to offload some of the burden on Accident and Emergency departments, to improve access to healthcare professionals and to help reduce GP workloads by providing treatment and information for minor conditions.

As with NHS Direct, walk-in centres have been subject to the criticism that they have not undergone formal assessment. In the initial period, 40 centres were opened in England. The King's Fund Report published at the end of 2001 has called for a halt in the expansion of the pilot programme, and has highlighted the need for more skills training for nurses and improved links with GPs and other healthcare providers. The next step is now awaited in the light of this report.

When trying to determine the efficacy of walk-in centres, it is worth bearing in mind that:

- they direct funds from other areas of primary care

- there can be a lack of continuity of care

- the service may generate a new demand.

○ (2002) An observational study comparing quality of care in walk-in centres with GP and NHS Direct using standardised patients. *BMJ*. **324**:1556–9.
This study looked at five clinical scenarios, namely postcoital contraception, chest pain, sinusitis, headache and asthma. Walk-in centres performed adequately and safely compared with GPs and NHS Direct for the above conditions. It was concluded that further research is needed on the impact of referrals on the workload of other healthcare providers.

○ (2003) Effect of NHS walk-in centres on local primary healthcare services: before and after observational study. *BMJ*. **326**: 530–2.
This study looked at the effect of a walk-in centre in Loughborough on local primary and emergency services. Market Harborough was used as the control town. It was found that the workload of GPs was not greatly affected. However, the minor injuries unit (attached to the walk-in centre) experienced a significant increase in workload.

○ (2003) Impact of NHS walk-in centres on workload of other healthcare providers: time series analysis. *BMJ*. **326**: 532–7.
This study was statistically inconclusive, but found a small increase in GP workload the year after the centre opened.

Intermediate care

'Intermediate care' is a new phrase for the old concept of bridging the gap between primary and secondary care. This is not just about providing social care for elderly patients in an effort to free hospital beds, but can also encompass various schemes, such as mental health, the young chronically ill, etc. It should not be regarded as a cheap alternative to acute hospital and specialist care.

Intermediate care, by definition, is not part of the current GP contract/GMS services. Although much of the medical input is provided by GPs, it does not follow that if no GP cover is available these patients should be allocated to a GP until they are discharged from their intermediate-care bed. It is envisaged that intermediate-care beds would primarily be nurse managed on a day-to-day basis, and GPs would be involved in the diagnostic, management and review aspects. It is a way for GPs to be involved and potentially influence the outpatient system.

The first trials of these plans were conducted in Leicester.

○ (1999) Randomized controlled trial of effectiveness of Leicester hospital-at-home scheme compared with hospital care. *BMJ.* **319**: 1542.
There was no significant difference at 3 months in mortality, change in health status or readmission rates in either the hospital-at-home group or the inpatient group.

○ (2000) Hospital at home vs. hospital care in patients with exacerbations of COPD: prospective randomised controlled trial. *BMJ.* **321**: 1245–8.
Again there was no difference in readmission rates, lung function or mortality at 3 months.

○ (2001) Stroke rehabilitation at home. *Age & Ageing.* **30**: 303–10.
This study looked at the effectiveness and cost of rehabilitation compared with follow-up in a day hospital. In a randomised controlled trial of 480 patients there was no difference in outcome or cost.

For intermediate care/hospital-at-home care to be successful, it is important to set up measurements of success, and to determine the types of patients who are to be cared for and the level of care to be input, as well as determining resource allocation. A new paper, *Intermediate Care and Specialist GPs*, calls for the expansion of the numbers of GPs and nurses with the necessary educational support to cope with what will become an increased demand.

Nurse practitioners

Nurse practitioners are playing an increasingly large role in the service provision of primary care. With the ongoing struggle to fill GP posts in some areas, nurse practitioners will continue to expand their role. The latter is varied, depending on the skills and experience of the nurse, but the main areas of input are disease prevention, health promotion, chronic disease management, immunisation (child and travel), smears and family planning. Management of minor illnesses, triage and prescribing are areas of ongoing development.

From the GP's perspective this addition to the team will hopefully reduce workload and improve access and satisfaction, as well as standards of care. GPs will have more time for 'serious' problems, and may be able to operate bigger lists.

Possible problems include the following.

• Nurses are not regulated, so who will be accountable? Will it be us as GPs?

• Is a two-tier system being introduced? Will GP recruitment suffer further because of this, particularly in inner cities?

• We may lose continuity of care as the GP.

• Nurses may misdiagnose rarer but serious conditions.

• GPs may start to lose their generalist role.

- Protocols and guidelines need to be developed. Who will write these? Will it be the GP?

- Nurses as a body are already overloaded trying to reach NSF targets, etc. Can we really expand their role further?

- Funding and training as well as interest/staffing are areas where needs have to be met.

○ (2000) Nurse management of patients with minor illnesses in general practice: a multicentre randomised controlled trial. *BMJ.* **320**:1038–43.
Following recruitment of nurses and a 3-month training period, there was a 2-month pilot study in which patients who asked for a GP appointment were randomly allocated to either a GP or a nurse. Nurse consultations lasted for 10 minutes and consultations with doctors for 8 minutes on average. Prescriptions were issued at similar rates. Around 73% of patients who were seen by a nurse had no doctor input. The study concluded that practice nurses offered an effective service for people with minor illnesses.

○ (2000) Randomised controlled trial comparing cost-effectiveness of GPs and nurse practitioners in primary care. *BMJ.* **320**: 1048–53.
Costs were found to be similar (i.e. there was no cost benefit to nurse practitioners at this point in time).

○ (2002) Systematic review of whether nurse practitioners working in primary care can provide equivalent care to doctors. *BMJ.* **324**: 819–23.
This review concluded that there would be higher levels of patient satisfaction and a high quality of care. It acknowledged the different pressures on nurses and doctors. It pointed out that the trials did not look at missed diagnoses (i.e. long-term follow-up etc.).

Pharmacists

The role of the pharmacist in primary care is also increasing. Community pharmacists are an under-used resource in the NHS, despite their level of training. The Government launched the first wave of its National Medicines Management Programme in October 2001. This project may help the Government to go some way towards reaching its NSF targets and meeting patient demand.

The pilot study involves 26 primary care groups where pharmacists can take on repeat prescribing (under protocols) and conduct medicine reviews for the over-65s and patients with chronic diseases. They can also be available in surgeries to give advice on medicines to GPs and patients.

The primary care groups involved will have a full-time project manager to help integration. The pilots themselves will be managed by the National Prescribing Centre and the National Primary Care Development Team.

○ (2000) Repeat prescribing: a role for the community pharmacists in controlling and monitoring repeat prescriptions. *Br J Gen Prac.* **50**: 271–5.
This study looked at conventional repeat prescribing vs. pharmacist-managed prescribing. It concluded that pharmacist management is feasible. It identifies problems that are not always seen by GPs (in terms of compliance, adverse drug reactions or interactions), and could make savings (up to 18%) in the drug bill (i.e. it would outweigh the cost of the pharmacist).

○ (2001) Randomised controlled trial of clinical medication review by a pharmacist of e
receiving repeat prescriptions in general practice. *BMJ*. **323**: 1340–3.
This trial concluded that a clinical pharmacist can conduct effective consultations with elderly
patients in general practice to review their drugs. These reviews resulted in changes in patients'
drugs and saved more than the cost of the intervention, without affecting the workload of GPs.

The British Lifestyle Survey 2001 (conducted by the consumer researcher Mintel) found that the number of people who asked the pharmacist for advice had increased by 25%. Over-the-counter analgesic sales have risen by 41%, and sales for remedies for coughs and colds have increased by 10%, all over the last 10 years.

Patient information leaflets (PIL) serve the medicolegal purpose of informing patients by listing all of the side-effects and contraindications of drugs. Although on the face of it this is a good thing, depending on the patient it can be counter-productive.

Personal Medical Services

Personal Medical Services (PMS) is an alternative to GMS (set out in the Red Book), and as yet is voluntary, although the NHS Plan 'expects' 30% of GPs to move to PMS by 2002, and all single-handers by 2004. Although the self-employed independent contractor status can continue, independence is being eroded.

PMS was actually introduced by the Conservative Government in the Primary Care Act 1997 after the initial concept had been introduced in *Choices and Opportunities*, a White Paper. It went live in April 1998 with a core contract that doctors had to fulfil. The contract is now to be scrapped in favour of a broad framework with outcomes and targets to be agreed locally.

The intention of PMS is to address local service issues and pilot new ways of delivering and improving services by allowing local flexibility. The emphasis is on local funding for local issues, which will hopefully attract GPs into areas with recruitment problems.

PMS covers what people would normally expect from GMS, but delivery can be different. The focus is on competitive services, achieving targets and a minimum of three audits per year. PMS providers will be accountable for delivery of National Service Frameworks and other key national clinical governance requirements (health improvement programmes, risk management, audits, workforce planning, etc.).

An Introduction to PMS is a GPC publication which covers the following aims of PMS:

● promoting persistently high-quality services

● providing opportunities and incentives for primary care professionals to use their skills to the full

● providing more flexible employment opportunities

● addressing recruitment and retention problems

- reducing the bureaucracy involved in the management of primary care provision.

As would be expected, PMS has had a variable reception. As happens with all new developments, the initial money available (especially for growth) was quite substantial, but this is no longer the case. Also, interestingly, the PMS core contract for third-wavers is much more directive.

The King's Fund study entitled *Current thoughts on PMS so far* was published in October 2001. It concluded by using the term 'disappointing'.

Personal Medical Services Pilots: Modernising Primary Care? states that 'there is little strong or consistent evidence of a "PMS effect" on quality'.

A PMS contract is not enforceable by law, but both parties are subject to binding arbitration by the Secretary of State for Health. It is thought that the aims of PMS could be achieved under the Red Book if it was updated. This is currently under way.

Benefits of PMS

- It is locally negotiated, and can reflect local circumstances.
- There is less management bureaucracy (e.g. item-of-service claims).
- There are flexible employment opportunities, with opportunities and incentives to develop skills.
- There is improved integration of the primary healthcare team.
- More services are available for patients.
- It addresses recruitment and retention problems in general practice.
- It promotes consistently high-quality services.
- It is practice based, not a contract with an individual doctor (i.e. illness, maternity leave, etc.). Much like the new GMS contract will be.

Drawbacks of PMS

- It is local, not national – so is not aligned with national pay reviews, and there is no agreement on pensions.
- There is annual renegotiation, and the contract is then fixed for a year, which compromises income.
- Local Medical Committee statutory levy is not automatically taken.
- It is not clear what will happen to PMS in the light of the proposed new contract.

Your contract, your future

www.bma.org.uk

The Red Book – our terms of service – has been renegotiated and costed, looking at the workload, infrastructure, practice expenses and skill-mix changes that will be necessary.

The contract will be between the primary care trust and the practice (i.e. there will be no individual lists), and will be for essential and additional services. The contract will safeguard premises, allowing for improvement and development in the interest of quality patient care.

Investing in general practice: the new GMS contract

The new GMS contract has been accepted and should:

- provide new mechanisms to allow practices greater flexibility to determine the range of services that they wish to provide

- reward practices for delivering clinical and organisational quality and for improving the patient's experience

- facilitate the modernisation of practice infrastructure, including premises and IT

- provide for unprecedented and guaranteed levels of investment through a gross investment guarantee

- support the delivery of a wider range of higher-quality services, and empower patients to make the best use of primary care services

- simplify the regulatory regime

- be implemented as soon as possible.

UK expenditure on primary care should rise from £6.1 billion to £8 billion over 3 years (a 31% increase).

More flexible provision of services

All GMS practices will provide essential services and a range of enhanced services. Practices will have the opportunity to increase their income by opting to provide a wider range of enhanced services.

Primary care organisations are responsible for ensuring that patient access is not compromised, and by 31 December 2004 they should have taken full responsibility for out-of-hours (6.30p.m.–8.00a.m. weekdays, all weekends, bank holidays and public holidays). This will include GP co-operatives, NHS Direct/24, walk-in centres, practice partnerships, paramedics, pharmacists, GP services in Accident and Emergency departments, commercial deputising services and social work services.

How will the money flow?

1 *Protected global sum*: paid directly to the practice from the primary care trust for essential and additional services, this represented much of the past Red Book payments.

2 *Enhanced services payments*: from the primary care organisation, includes development money.

3 *Wisdom and experience payments*: from the primary care organisation, for more senior doctors.

4 *Quality and outcome payments*:
   - infrastructure (e.g. premises, IT, staff)
   - aspiration (declared by the practice at the beginning of the year)
   - reward (paid at the end of the year if aspirations are met).

Categorisation of services

Essential services

These are provided by every practice, and the service is initiated by the patient. They include the following:

- management of patients who are ill:
  - relevant health promotion
  - appropriate referral

- general management of patients who are terminally ill

- chronic disease management.

Addition services

Most practices would be expected to provide these, but could opt out if necessary (e.g. because of staff shortages):

- cervical screening

- contraceptive services

- vaccinations and immunisations (target payments of 70% and 90% respectively remain)

- child health surveillance

- maternity services (intrapartum care would be an enhanced service)

- minor surgery.

Enhanced services

These are essential or additional services delivered to a higher specific standard, as well as innovative services. They will allow primary care organisations to invest in areas such as routine home visits, patient transport, services for violent patients, etc.

There will be:

- national direction with specifications and benchmark pricing which all primary care organisations must commission
- national minimum specifications and benchmark pricing that are not directed
- local development.

Breadth of care will be rewarded through holistic care payments.

This categorisation would allow GPs to:

- control their workload
- receive guaranteed resources
- opt out of additional services if they are unable to provide them
- offer innovative services.

New services will only ever be introduced when the necessary additional resources have been provided. GPs will have a choice as to whether to provide out-of-hours care. If they do not want to do so, then the primary care trust carries the responsibility for providing this care.

Rewarding quality and outcomes

The quality framework will have four main components focusing on four domains each with key indicators.

1 *Clinical standards (10 areas)*: coronary heart disease, stroke or transient ischaemic attack, hypertension, diabetes, chronic obstructive pulmonary disease, epilepsy, cancer, mental health, hypothyroidism and asthma.

2 *Organisational standards (5 areas)*: records and information about patients, information for patients, education and training, medicines management and clinical and practice management.

3 *Experience of patients (2 areas)*: covering the services provided, how they are provided and their involvement in service development plans; this will include survey consultation length.

4 *Additional services (4 areas)*: cervical screening, child health surveillance, maternity services and contraceptive services.

At the beginning of the year, the practice will receive a proportion of the quality payment for the standard aspired to – the *aspiration payment*. Once the standard has been achieved, the practice will receive the remainder – the *achievement payment*. There will also be (in the first 3 years only) *preparation payment*.

Exception reporting will be in place to ensure that practices do not lose payment as a result of factors beyond their control. Similarly, certain categories of patient will be excluded (e.g. those who are terminally ill, those on maximum medication, newly diagnosed patients, etc.).

As part of this original document, global sum payments were to be calculated using the Carr–Hill allocation formula. However, there were problems with the weighting of this, especially for practices with accurate practice lists. The allocation formula for the global sum will now be applied to the registered practice population from 1 April 2004. As a result of this and concerns about income, a *minimum practice income guarantee (MPIG)* for the first few years has been confirmed. The formula data are now under full review following the 'yes' vote.

○ (2002) A fresh new contract for GPs. *BMJ*. **324**: 1048–9.

'Currently allocation of resources only poorly reflects patients' needs. It focuses on individual GPs and fails to recognise the role of the practice team. Quality measures are sparse and crudely applied and perverse incentives often serve to reward poor-quality services.'

National pricing of the new contract (announced on 19 April 2002) will take into account changing demands on primary care through an annual assessment of workload. If the workload rises, new resources will be made available.

In the future, GPs will be better able to control their workload. Furthermore, incentives for GPs will change (i.e. there will be more focus on quality).

NHS Cancer Plan

This was introduced in September/October 2000 following a series of cancer guidelines, the aim being to improve cancer care and outcome in the NHS. The plan was developed by a multidisciplinary team, but for it to have any impact it will need 'local leadership and support'. Each primary care trust will have a cancer lead.

The Government will play its part by investing in the workforce and tackling shortages. There will be 1000 new cancer specialists, and histopathology, radiography and nursing will also be targeted.

It is hoped that the plan will be achieved by increasing capacity through new ways of working and developing opportunities, as well as by education, recruitment and retention planning. Needless to say, a variety of opinions have been expressed in editorials and in the letters pages, ranging from 'excellent, simple, clear, GP and patient centred' to 'a waste of money, politically motivated and barely enough investment to keep up with the increasing incidence of cancer'.

The plan has four aims:

1 to save more lives

2 to ensure that people with cancer receive professional support and care as well as the best treatment

3 to tackle inequalities in health which mean that unskilled workers are twice as likely to die from cancer as professionals

4 to build a future through cancer research and preparation for a genetic revolution.

There are three new commitments:

1 to reduce smoking in manual workers from 32% (in 1998) to 26% by 2010

2 to reduce waiting times for diagnosis and treatment to 1 month (from an urgent cancer referral to starting treatment) by 2005

3 to invest an extra £50 million in hospices and specialist palliative care.

Also discussed is the role of promoting a healthier diet – the 'five-a-day' programme. As well as raising public awareness, children aged 4–6 years will be able to have a piece of fruit every day if they wanted. (It is unclear how this is going to work. Will it be offered at lunch for dessert?)

There are plans to extend cancer screening.

- *Breast cancer sreening*: will be extended to women aged 65–70 by 2004, and available on request to those over 70 years of age.

- *Cervical screening*: the programme will be upgraded and unnecessary repeats reduced.

- *Colorectal cancer*: pilots are now completed and under discussion. If they are successful, population screening for those aged 50–69 years will be introduced.

- *Prostate cancer*: prostate-specific antigen (PSA) tests will be available to empower men to make their own choices. No formal programme is planned, as too many questions remain unanswered.

- *Ovarian cancer*: trials are in progress.

Finally, there will be investment in research, in particular the National Cancer Research Institute. Advances in genetics will lead to a greater understanding of inherited susceptibility in the future. As things stand, the cancer genetics service needs a strategic framework to develop further. The Harper Report recommended that primary care should be the principal focus for clinical cancer genetics. This in turn came from the Calman–Hine Report, which recommended that there should be networks of cancer care in research, assessment, diagnosis and treatment.

National Institute for Clinical Excellence (NICE)

www.nice.org.uk

NICE was launched in England and Wales in 1999 with the following aims:

- to produce national guidelines on individual technologies (including drugs)

- to produce clinical guidelines on the management of specific conditions

- to encourage improvement by the use of audit.

It exists to produce guidelines for health professionals and must ensure that its advice is based on rigorous analysis of all of the available evidence, both clinical and economic. Its decisions are advisory, not mandatory.

As part of NICE there is a Referral Practice Project Steering Group, which is responsible for the recently published guidelines.

Following the controversial reversal of its decision on Zanamivir, since April 2001 all evidence has had to be open. However, there are still concerns that NICE may be influenced by industry or patient organisations.

○ (2001) Wrong SIGN, NICE mess: is national guidance distorting allocation of resources? *BMJ.* **323**: 743–5.
   This article discusses the Scottish Intercollegiate Guidelines Network (SIGN) and NICE. The authors state that the way forward to remedy some of the problems is for NICE to become a recognised rationing agency. It should say no to relatively costly and ineffective new drugs. The authors suggest implementing a fixed growth budget for new technologies, distributed to primary care trusts.

○ (2000) The failings of NICE. *BMJ.* **321**: 1363.
   This editorial was written in the early days, criticising NICE (and politicians) for not admitting to their role of rationing within the NHS.

○ (2002) From guidance to practice: why NICE is not enough. *BMJ.* **324**: 842–5.
   This article suggests that NICE will only work if the Health Service supports and implements the changes that it promotes. At present this is not the case.

There was a question on the differences between implicit and explicit rationing in the MRCGP exam in 2000. It is thought that NICE will encourage implicit rationing by delay (waiting lists, discrimination among the elderly and the mentally ill) and dilution (of specialist care) (e.g. two nurses instead of four on an elderly-care ward to cover the drug costs). This was part of the reason why the authors of the 'NICE mess' article cited above felt that NICE should also be able to refuse to give guidance on some areas if it felt that it was appropriate to do so.

The House of Commons Health Committee has conducted an inquiry into NICE (January 2002). This considered to what extent the institute has provided independent, clear and credible guidance, and also whether it has enabled patients to have quicker access to drugs that are known to be effective, and whether guidance is accepted locally and acted upon. The Health Select Committee and the Consumers' Association have criticised the work of NICE as flaws have been found in the guidance issued.

National Service Frameworks

NSFs were proposed in the 1998 White Paper *A First-Class Service: Quality in the New NHS* as part of the Government's agenda to drive up quality and reduce unacceptable variations in health and social services across the UK. They have been proposed as accompaniments to NICE and identified as priorities in *Modernising Health and Social Services: National Priorities Guidance for 1999/2000–2000/01.*

The standards will be set by NICE and NSFs, delivered by clinical governance and underpinned by self-regulation and lifelong learning. The Commission for Health Improvement, the National Performance Assessment Framework and the National Survey of Patients will be used to monitor the NSFs. Performance will be assessed by means of a small number of national milestones and high-level performance indicators.

There will be advances and changes during the implementation of the NSFs. Therefore they will have to evolve if they are to remain relevant and credible in such a changing environment. Similarly, the need for learning and development (organisational, professional and personal) is recognised.

Objectives of NSFs

These are as follows:

1 to address the problems that affect quality of NHS care
2 to tackle variations in:
   - agreed standards of care
   - data collection and audit
   - local provision of national services
   - funding and resources
   - involvement with non-NHS agencies.

Personal development plans

The need for personal development plans (PDPs) has been recognised and evolved from the shortcomings of 30 hours of undirected Postgraduate Educational Allowance (PGEA), as well as media attention that has focused on recent medical scandals (e.g. the Bristol Inquiry and the Shipman case). Revalidation will require us to demonstrate our learning, which we will have to map out according to our own individual needs. These will in turn be determined by priorities which are dictated by the influences around us, namely national influences, primary care groups, and practice and personal needs.

Good Medical Practice in General Practice, published by the Royal College of General Practitioners, states that an excellent GP:

- is up to date and regularly reviews their knowledge

- uses these reviews to develop practice and their personal development plan

- uses a range of methods to monitor and meet their educational needs.

A First-Class Service: Quality in the New NHS is a 1998 Government publication which states that lifelong learning will give NHS staff the knowledge necessary to offer the most effective and high-quality care to patients. Continuous professional development programmes need to meet the learning needs of the individual, inspire public confidence in their skills, and also meet the wider developmental needs of the NHS.

The *NHS Plan*, which was published in July 2000, is about staff working 'smarter not harder'! All doctors employed within the NHS have been required to participate in annual appraisals and clinical audit since 2001.

The advantages of personal development can be summarised as follows:

- personal satisfaction
- personally relevant
- more flexible
- aspirations are achieved
- helps reflection
- fulfils contract requirements
- improved patient care
- more cost-effective
- no PGEA.

The disadvantages can be summarised as follows:

- can lead to isolation
- loss of objectivity
- may be overwhelming
- needs support network/mentor
- need more time investment
- may be reinforcing skills that are adequate

PGEA hours will eventually be obtainable through the PDP process, until they are abandoned. The speed with which this happens and exactly how it will be assessed will depend upon the region.

Writing a PDP/practice development plan

In addition to a PDP, when working in a GP setting/partnership there will be a requirement for a practice development plan. This is based on the same principles as a PDP.

Identifying learning needs

These represent the gap between the way things are now and the way they should be or how you want them to be in the future. Learning needs can be identified by keeping lists, reviewing referrals, conducting audits, significant event analysis, asking colleagues, etc. (known as the 'Johari window').

Setting learning objectives and measure of success

Objectives may involve knowledge, skills, attitudes etc. Success can be looked at by reflection, feedback, audit, reduction in demand, etc.

Identifying resource implications and time scales

This means that plans should be achievable.

Seeking evidence of achievement

A formal PDP is one stage of a continuous process. The evidence can be used to make a *learning portfolio* (i.e. a long-term record of past experience and future aspirations) containing workload logs, case descriptions, videos, audits, patient surveys, reflection, significant event analysis, etc. This is the 'cradle to grave' idea.

Although the plan has now been formalised, conscientious doctors have already been doing this for years, as it is the fundamental principle that underpins adult learning, educational theories and learning cycles. We all want to develop and work within an effective team, improve clinical care, plan constructively and provide mechanisms of accountability. PDPs are a starting point for this which will also help us to bid for resources in the future.

Revalidation: professional self-regulation

www.revalidationuk.info
www.appraisaluk.info

With persistent negative media attention, fuelled by the Bristol Inquiry and the Harold Shipman case, it is understandable that the public are finding it increasingly difficult to have faith in their doctors and the General Medical Council (GMC). Partly because of this, the GMC is undergoing a period of reform aimed mainly at proving that it is capable of regulating the profession. However, the responsibility for basic competence is that of the individual doctor – it always has been and always will be. One of the difficulties that has been highlighted by various editorials is how to make revalidation stimulating and worthwhile for the majority of doctors while at the same time sensitive enough to pick out those who are performing poorly.

Revalidation: the Privileges and Obligations of Registration is one of the documents that cover this (it can be downloaded from www.gmc-uk.org). The GMC sees the benefits in terms of those for patients, doctors and employers. It makes the register valid in terms of fitness to practise, and promotes good medical practice while protecting against poorly performing doctors. It will also help to protect doctors from unfounded criticisms, as they will be able to show that they are giving good medical care.

Revalidation for Clinical General Practice was produced by a revalidation party for the Royal College of General Practitioners. It anticipates that revalidation will be related to a number of different systems (e.g. clinical governance, accredited professional development, appraisal, GMC performance procedures, etc).

The criteria they have identified for revalidation to work are as follows.

- It should be understood by the public and be credible.

- It should identify unacceptable performance.

- It should identify good performance.

- It should be supported by the profession and support the profession.

- It should be practical and feasible.

- It should not put any GPs or practices at an advantage or disadvantage.

Revalidation should be a continuous process with an episode submission and assessment of fitness to practise having been through an annual appraisal process.

The initial 500 revalidation pilot forms have been a self-reported success. The claim is that the form should take about 6 hours to complete, it will consist of three sections, and will be appraised annually by another medical practitioner who is accountable to the GMC. Every 5 years a revalidation group will assess the folder. These plans have all yet to be finalised.

A Licence to Practise and Revalidation – GMC April 2003

Copies of this document can be downloaded from publications@gmc-uk.org.

The register will be strengthened by a new system based on licence to practise, supported by periodic revalidation. This will be based on the GMC's *Good Medical Practice* and can be done through the appraisal route or, if you have not had an appraisal by April 2005, the independent route.

- In 2004, new GMC fee arrangements will be announced, and all doctors will be issued with a licence to practise.

- In 2005, revalidation will start (invitation will be random).

The proposed layout for the folder is as follows:

- *Section 1: Personal registration details* – also providing a contact address.

- *Section 2: What you do* – information about your field of practice, actual activities and time spent on them each week.

- *Section 3: Information and data about your practice*
  - audit and results
  - critical incidents – your role and the changes made
  - structured reviews and surveys of your practice by other professionals

- routine indicators (PACT data, admissions etc.)
- investigations by, for example, the Royal College of General Practitioners and the National Clinical Assessment Authority, and their results
- details of articles and books published, as well as qualifications gained
- subscriptions to professional journals
- your role in producing guidelines and protocols
- PGEA totals
- complaints and resulting changes
- training and teaching roles
- details of your own health problems or convictions
- disciplinary action by an employer
- confirmation that you have not knowingly withheld any relevant information.

This process has been talked about for years, but has not occurred until now because of lack of interest and resources. If we do not take on the responsibility now, as a profession, it will be done for us. 'Self-regulation is a privilege, not a right.'

Accredited professional development

This is a new scheme designed by the Royal College of General Practitioners and the Medical Defence Union as a joint initiative. It will consist of six work modules taken over 5 years that are designed to facilitate learning in a way that will be relevant to everyday general practice (i.e. not just for the purpose of revalidation). The module 'keeping up to date and improving care' is ongoing, while the remaining five are estimated to take 6 to 12 months each.

Essential areas that are covered include the following:

- personal (e.g. special interests)

- professional – maintaining up-to-date knowledge in line with *Good Medical Practice for GPs*

- practice-based issues

- health service priorities (e.g. NSFs).

In addition, the scheme covers the GMC's seven broad areas of practice:

- good clinical care

- maintaining good clinical practice

- relationships with patients

- working with colleagues

- teaching and training

- probity – attention to the ethics and science of research

- health.

The toolkit can be download from www.rcgp.org.uk/rcgp/quality_unit/toolkit/index.asp

Clinical governance

www.cgsupport.org (clinical governance support website).

Whereas revalidation is a professional-based measure to ensure high standards of care, clinical governance has more of a management basis, being accountable to the Government through the primary care trust/primary care groups. It is aimed at 'improving the quality of services offered in the NHS and safeguarding high standards' as well as 'creating an environment in which clinical excellence will flourish'.

It was published in a Labour Government White Paper to highlight to the public the fact that the NHS will not tolerate anything less than the best. This is to be achieved in a no-blame, questioning, learning culture.

In 1999, an NHS Clinical Governance Support Team was established to support the development and implementation of clinical governance. This team is now part of the Modernisation Agency. NICE will develop guidelines for the standards expected of general practitioners.

The Commission for Health Improvement (which consists of GPs, community nurses and lay people) is a PCG-based group. Its function is to look at clinical governance in practices and to try to effect necessary change. It will visit each PCG every 4 years and select practices at random. It can report directly to the Health Secretary if necessary.

The Government has done for medicine what it did for teaching, and created *beacon practice* status for those deemed to be 'most worthy'. These practices demonstrate high standards of access, patient care, health improvement, etc. They are paid a nominal £4000 per year, and in return are expected to promote their way of working, mainly through 12 open days per year at the practice.

Each GP has a responsibility to provide a high quality of care and to audit this. At present GP care is too variable (this in itself has advantages and disadvantages), and patients need to be confident that their doctor is up to date and offering effective treatment. Clinical governance is an effective tool for monitoring and improving quality of care in general practice.

○ (2001) Implementing clinical governance. *BMJ*. **322**: 1413–17.
This article gives a brief overview of evolution and the key elements of NHS quality strategy.

○ (2001) Improving the quality of care through clinical governance. *BMJ*. **322**: 1580–2.
This is the third part of the series in the *BMJ*. One of the main obstacles envisaged is limited resources. This is followed by a slow pace of change.

○ (2002) The role of clinical governance as a strategy for quality improvement in primary care. *Br J Gen Pract*. **52(Suppl. 1)**: S12–17.
This paper considers the process of implementing clinical governance in primary care and its impact on quality improvement. It states that success for implementation requires a multi-level approach to change (GP, primary care trust and NHS) and also that there are three overlapping sets of issues which enhance implementation, namely the environment (context), the leaders and the implementers/users of the change. The whole of this supplement is on quality.

Significant event analysis

This process is known by various names, including significant event audit, critical event audit or analysis, and significant event review. It can involve examples of when things go right as well as when they go wrong. It can be clinical or non-clinical, and it can involve anyone in the team, the point being that such events are powerful motivators for change, and the questions that may be raised could identify a previously unidentified learning need. Significant event analysis should be felt to be a positive experience by all those involved.

How can significant event analysis be organised?

- Decide who is to be involved (e.g. doctors, nurses, receptionists, administration/office staff).
- How are they to be involved (regular meetings, triggered by specific cases)?
- The time interval after the event should not be too long, otherwise momentum is lost and details are forgotten.
- It should be free of interruptions.
- A suitable environment is needed. Does it need to be outside the workplace?
- Set ground rules (e.g. with regard to confidentiality and anonymity).
- Appoint a chairperson and scribe for appropriate record keeping.
- The agenda should cover the following questions.
  - Why has the significant event been chosen?
  - What do people want to achieve by analysing it?
  - What are the facts of the case? (These are often circulated before the meeting.)
  - What issues are raised (e.g. care, communication)?
  - What went well?
  - What went badly and how can things be improved? Any shortcomings that are highlighted should be things that are amenable to change, rather than personal attacks, and comments should be constructive.
  - What action should be taken?
    - (i)   Formulate a plan.
    - (ii) Prioritise points.
    - (iii) Decide upon a time scale.
    - (iv) Consider how success can be determined.

Medical error

> To err is human.

Around 100 000 people die each year in the USA as a result of iatrogenic causes. Reducing medical mishaps is fundamental to improving quality. 'First do no harm' is part of our Hippocratic oath. Harm is done every day, and it needs skill to translate these negative events into useful information. For this to happen there needs to be some type of reporting to enable system changes which will improve patient safety.

Doctors tend to overestimate their ability to function flawlessly under adverse conditions such as fatigue, time pressure and high anxiety. Aviation and other non-medical 'hands-on' industries have developed incident reporting where the focus is on *near misses*. There are incentives for voluntary reporting, confidentiality is ensured, and the emphasis is on data collection, analysis and improvement, rather than the old-style punitive approach.

Gaps in continuity of care that lead to near misses or harm can occur at three levels, namely individual people, stages or processes. Increasing safety can be achieved by understanding and reinforcing our ability to bridge these gaps. Despite all of the defences, barriers and safeguards that are inbuilt, mistakes will continue to occur, so the aim should be to minimise the risks at each stage.

For example, system changes that would improve patient safety would include the following:

- reducing complexity

- optimising information processing

- automating wisely (i.e. using IT to support human operation rather than because it is available)

- using constraints to restrict certain actions

- mitigating the unwanted side-effects of change (e.g. testing on a small scale, trying to predict problems and monitor the outcome).

Examples where this approach has been successful are seen in the pharmaceutical industry with drugs and anaesthetic attachments.

Virtually a whole issue of the *British Medical Journal* (18 March 2000) was dedicated to medical error. The 'error prevention movement' has accelerated, and major changes are occurring in the way that we think about and carry out our daily work. There is an undercurrent of more slowly evolving cultural change in our learning, responsibilities and ability to admit fallibility.

For *risk assessment* (i.e. reporting of near misses) to be successful, incidents need to be analysed in an organisational way rather than on a personal basis. Formal protocols need to be developed to ensure systematic, comprehensive and efficient investigations. As always, training needs to be part of the developing programme if it is to be a standardised and effective tool.

○ (2003) Acknowledgement of 'no fault' medical injury: review of patients' hospital records in New Zealand. *BMJ*. **326**: 79–80.
  This review reported that doctors in counties with a no-fault compensation system for medical injuries were more likely to report mistakes.

Should systems reporting be voluntary?

An example of voluntary reporting is the Safe Medical Devices Act 1990. Reporting is fundamental to the broad goal of error reduction. *Non-punitive, confidential, voluntary* reporting programmes provide more useful information about errors and their causes than mandatory reporting for the following reasons.

- There is no fear of retribution.

- The depth of information is the key to understanding the problem. If reporting is forced, then the primary motivation is self-protection and adherence to requirement, *not* to help others to avoid making the same mistake.

In the *BMJ* issue referred to earlier in this section (18 March 2000), a number of papers and editorials highlighted the need to move away from individual blame towards an organisational approach where we acknowledge that mistakes are inevitable. By doing this, we can build systems to prevent such events occurring and have a means of identifying them early on (i.e. moving away from the *personal approach* towards a *systems approach*).

However, as things change in the future in the name of *continuous quality improvement*, it must be remembered that the person who makes the mistake needs help, too (a point that is all too easy to forget and which is often overlooked).

○ (2002) Learning from adverse incidents involving medical devices. *BMJ*. **325**: 272–5.
   The NHS is perceived to have a poor record of learning from incidents, despite the efforts of the Medical Devices Agency to issue safety warnings. This study found that adverse incidents were typically caused by alignment of different factors, but that good practice can prevent errors from becoming incidents.

National Clinical Assessment Authority

This was established in April 2001 as part of the Government's commitment to quality, its purpose being to investigate and assist doctors if necessary to resolve problems in performance at an early stage when they have been unable to resolve them at a local level. Such doctors are referred to the National Clinical Assessment Authority either by their employers or by themselves, *not* by patients.

There may be some overlap with the Commission for Health Improvement.

Assessments will all be confidential, the exception being where a statutory power (e.g. the police or the General medical Council) requires information.

National Patient Safety Agency

The role of the National Patient Safety Agency (NPSA) is to promote an open and fair reporting culture, collecting, collating, categorising and coding adverse incidents, looking for patterns and trends, and acting on identified risk.

The NPSA was established in July 2001 to improve patient safety by running a national reporting system to log adverse clinical events and near misses, so that lessons could be shared and learned from in a blame-free way.

GPs have to report all incidents in which a patient was or could have been seriously harmed.

This follows the publication of a document entitled *A Commitment to Quality, a Quest for Excellence* in June 2001.

The NPSA document *Doing Less Harm* applies the reporting rule to all incidents, including anaphylaxis and unexpected death in the surgery, both of which are categorised as 'red'. Other incidents will be categorised as green, yellow or orange, depending on their severity.

Commission for Health Improvement

This is a body representing the Government which is made up of GPs, nurses and lay people who look at clinical governance at a primary care group (PCG) level every 4 years. They can report under-performing PCGs to the Health Secretary, and they will mainly investigate organisational systems.

New proposals are being suggested in the NHS Reform and Health Care Professions Bill where the Commission for Health Improvement (CHI) will be able to recommend that the Health Secretary takes 'special measures' against failing GP practices. This new bill will also create an office within the CHI to collect and publish statistics on primary care services and give patient groups the right to inspect all general practice premises.

Primary care groups

PCGs were set up on 1 April 1999, working with patients and health authority representatives to develop healthcare needs in local communities following the publication of the Government's White Paper *The New NHS: Modern, Dependable*.

The aim is that PCGs will ultimately develop trust status and take over from the health authority.

There are four levels of PCG, depending on responsibility.

- Level 1 – supports the health authority in commissioning.

- Level 2 – develops budget responsibility.

- Level 3 – free-standing body accountable to the health authority for commissioning (i.e. primary care trust).

- Level 4 – as for Level 3, but also covers provision of community services.

A *primary care trust* (PCT) is run by its board and the PCT Professional Executive Committee (PEC). The board itself consists of three heads who are responsible for strategic planning:

- the chief executive, usually an NHS manager

- the PCT chairman, a lay person appointed by the Appointments Commission

- the PEC chairman, usually a GP.

There is a medical director (who is not usually on the board) who is responsible for the day-to-day running of the clinical services.

Medical/clinical audit

Audit definitions have evolved somewhat, from Maurin's 1976 thoughts (in terms of it being a general counting exercise) to the modern-day Government's description in *Working for Patients*, which defines audit as: 'the systematic critical analysis of the quality of medical care, including procedures used for diagnosis and treatment, the use of resources and the resulting outcome and quality of life for the patients' (i.e. it is a much more active approach).

Three major categories have been identified by Donabedian (1982):

1 Audit of *structure* – delivery of care (e.g. appointments)

2 Audit of *process* – how patients are treated (e.g. looking at prescriptions)

3 Audit of *outcome* – what ultimately happens (e.g. mortality, morbidity).

In *Duties of a Doctor* the General Medical Council describes audit as an essential professional responsibility. The Royal College of General Practitioners Information Service published an information leaflet on medical audit in March 2001. A copy of this can be downloaded from www.rcgp.org.uk.

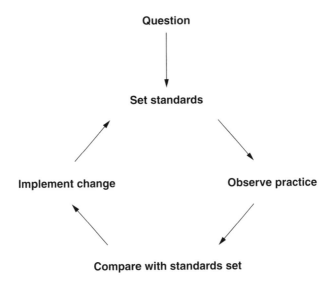

Summary of the audit cycle

Audit is a means by which we can look systematically and critically at our work – it is the final stage of evidence-based medicine. It is not research (research is done to find out what best practice is). Audit is a measure of performance against a predetermined standard. It can highlight problems, encourage change, reduce errors and demonstrate good care.

Audit is increasingly part of clinical governance, and will become an integral part of revalidation. Help with audits can be found in primary care audit groups and medical audit advisory groups.

Complaints

A complaint is an expression of dissatisfaction that requires a response. The number of complaints against GPs has doubled in the last 10 years. Handling complaints well puts things right for the individual who has received a poor service, and it also allows those services to be improved. Resolving complaints at an early stage is the ultimate aim.

The main complaints encountered in general practice are as follows:

- delayed diagnosis, failure to make a diagnosis, or an incorrect diagnosis

- failure to visit

- surgery appointment times/availability

- staff attitudes/rudeness

- inadequate examination

- refusal to refer.

The majority of complaints are related to GMS paragraph 13 (provision of services to patients).

If an individual wishes to make a complaint, this should ideally be done within 6 months of the incident, or within 6 months of finding out that there was something to complain about. The general consensus is that a complaint should be made within 1 year.

The *NHS complaints procedure* has three stages:

1 local resolution (with or without an independent lay conciliator liaising between the two parties)

2 a convenor, who can request an independent review or refer back for local resolution

3 the ombudsman (Health Service Commissioner).

Complaints procedure in primary care

Following the publication of the Wilson Report *Being Heard* in 1994, the complaints procedure was revised in 1996, and it is now in the process of being updated again following the publication of a response document, *Reforming the NHS Complaints Procedure: a Listening Document*, which can be downloaded from: www.doh.gov.uk/nhscomplaintsreform.

All practices should have a written and publicised complaints procedure explaining who patients should speak to and what to expect. This is required as part of the terms of service. In the event of a complaint:

1 the nominated person or deputy should 'interview' the complainant and again explain the procedure

2 complaints must be acknowledged within two working days, or at the time if they are verbal

3 the complainant should receive a written response within 10 working days (or 20 working days if it is a hospital complaint). This response should:
   (i)   summarise the complaint
   (ii)   explain the patient's view of the complaint
   (iii)   apologise if this is appropriate
   (iv)   describe the outcome and steps taken
   (v)   explain the next step, and how to contact the health authority/primary care group if the patient is still unhappy.

Ensure that if the complaint is made by someone other than the patient, consent is obtained. Be clear and concise, and try to avoid medical terminology. If you do use medical terms, explain them clearly.

Practices should:

• keep separate complaints file

• include complaints statistics in the annual report, and for revalidation in the future

• hold practice meetings on complaints and how to manage them.

The NHS complaints procedure is not about taking disciplinary action, which would need to be investigated by a professional disciplinary body after having been referred by the health authority/primary care group to a disciplinary panel. Disciplinary measures can only be taken if a GP has failed to comply with his or her terms of service. Furthermore, the procedure does not deal with claims for financial compensation, private healthcare treatment or events about which an individual is already taking legal action.

The Independent Complaints Advocacy Service is the NHS body that will help patients or families who wish to lodge a complaint against the NHS.

Current issues

The Commission for Health Improvement is advocating a new complaints system which would allow under-performing GPs to be identified relatively quickly.

The main recommendation are as follows:

- anonymous complaints to be logged
- patients to be given more say in the appointment of new partners
- improved patient information about what to expect from the doctor–patient relationship.

The other main point that is being reviewed is local resolution, in that patients have to complain to their practice and cannot at their choosing bypass this in order to avoid unpleasantness and the possibility of being struck off the list (i.e. the possibility of dysfunctional relationships developing).

Consent

The *Reference Guide to Consent for Examination or Treatment* is a 30-page document produced by the Department of Health's 'Good Practice in Consent Advisory Group', which summarises legal requirements and good practice requirements on consent. *12 Key Points on Consent: the Law in England*, which was circulated to GPs, is available at www.doh.gov.uk/consent.

The document is relevant to all healthcare professionals, including students. It does not cover consent issues for the use of organs or tissues after death, nor does it include participation in observational studies or the use of personal information.

It is worth noting that the law changes depending on the different test cases that are brought. In addition, the European Human Rights Act will probably have some effect on English law.

The BMA ethics department published the *Consent Tool Kit* booklet in March 2000, which is aimed at improving understanding and the practice of obtaining valid consent. Similarly, the General Medical Council has published *Seeking Patients' Consent: the Ethical Considerations* and *Good Medical Practice*. The first of these covers the issues of consent, while the second raises awareness of the importance of consent in everyday practice.

The approach taken to consent is fundamental to the doctor–patient relationship, and highlights an individual's ethical viewpoint on a patient's autonomy. Tony Hope wrote a helpful ethically based article on consent in *Medicine* in October 2000. He suggests a quick three-point check on legal validity.

1 Is the patient properly informed?

2 Is the patient competent to give consent?

3 Did the patient give consent voluntarily (without coercion)?

From a legal point of view, consent provides the patient with a power of veto. Without consent, a patient could successfully sue a doctor for battery. Technically, touching another person without their consent constitutes battery (i.e. the patient does not need to have suffered harm). Similarly, a doctor could be found negligent if he or she has not given the patient certain relevant information to allow that patient to give informed consent.

The fact that a person comes to see a doctor or is admitted to hospital does not imply consent to any examination, investigation or treatment. In giving/refusing consent, it is important that the patient understands the reasons behind treatment, the associated risks and benefits, and the consequences if they refuse treatment. It does not matter how the patient gives consent. It can be written, verbal or non-verbal. A signature does not prove that consent is valid. Documentation of information given and consent is important.

Confidentiality

The success of the doctor–patient relationship is dependent on a number of factors. Confidentiality ('secrecy and discretion') has a therapeutically significant role, and has been fundamental to our code of practice since before the Hippocratic oath. Without its assurance, patients may be reluctant to give doctors the information that they need in order to provide good care. Information that is learned about a patient belongs to that patient (even after their death), and they have the right to determine who has access to it.

GMC Guidelines on confidentiality: protecting and providing information

These provide information on confidentiality and the holding and disclosing of information. These guidelines do not have the force of law, but are taken seriously by the courts.

Disclosure to a third party

A doctor's legal obligation of confidentiality is best seen as a public rather than a private interest (i.e. the obligation is not absolute, and in some situations the law allows or even obliges doctors to breach confidentiality).

Examples of circumstances where a doctor must breach confidentiality include termination of pregnancy (Abortion Act 1967), notifiable diseases (1984 Act), drug addiction (1973 Drug Misuse Act), births and deaths (Births, Deaths and Registration Act 1953), and forms for incapacity benefit. Police can request names and addresses (but not clinical details) of individuals who are alleged to be guilty under the Road Traffic Accident Act (1988).

Examples of circumstances where doctors have discretion to breach confidentiality include imparting information to other members of the healthcare team, a patient driving who is not fit to do so (the GMC advises informing the DVLA), and a third party being at significant risk (e.g. the partner of an HIV-positive patient).

Consent and confidentiality go hand in hand, and it is good practice to seek the patient's consent to disclosure of any information wherever possible, whether or not you judge that the patient can be identified from the disclosure.

The Data Protection Act 1998 requires everyone who processes personal information about living individuals to notify the Government Commissioner for Data Protection.

Access to Health Records Act (1990)

A patient has the right to see his or her medical records, obtain copies of these records and have the records explained.

Limitations include the following.

- This act only applies to records made after 1 November 1991. Records made before this date are included if they are needed to understand later notes.

- A doctor can deny access to a patient's medical records if he or she believes that serious harm to the patient's physical or mental health will result from seeing those records.

- The doctor should ensure that the confidentiality of other individuals is maintained.

Doctor's duties

- The doctor should enable the patient to see the records (or copies of them) within 21 days, or 40 days for records that are more than 40 days old.

- He or she can charge a reasonable fee for copying and time spent explaining records.

- He or she should make appropriate corrections if the original data are incorrect.

The Caldicott Report

The Caldicott Report was issued following the review of patient-identifiable information by the Caldicott Committee in December 1997.

The report was commissioned in the light of the publication of *The Protection and Use of Patient Information* in 1996, due to concerns about the way in which patient information is used in the NHS and the need to ensure that confidentiality is not undermined.

There are 16 recommendations (www.doh.gov.uk/confiden/crep.htm):

1 Every data flow, whether current or proposed, should be tested against basic principles of good practice. Continuing flows should be retested regularly.
2 A programme of work should be established to reinforce awareness of confidentiality and information security requirements among all staff within the NHS.
3 A senior person, preferably a health professional, should be nominated in each health organisation to act as a guardian who is responsible for safeguarding the confidentiality of patient information.
4 Clear guidance should be provided for those individuals/bodies responsible for approving uses of patient-identifiable information.
5 Protocols should be developed to protect the exchange of patient-identifiable information between NHS and non-NHS bodies.

6 The identity of those responsible for monitoring the sharing and transfer of information within agreed local protocols should be clearly communicated.

7 An accreditation system which recognises those organisations that are following good practice with respect to confidentiality should be considered.

8 The NHS number should replace all other identifiers wherever this is practicable, taking account of the consequences of errors and particular requirements for other specific identifiers.

9 Strict protocols should define who is authorised to gain access to patient identity where the NHS number or other coded identifier is used.

10 In cases where particularly sensitive information is transferred, privacy-enhanced technologies (e.g. encrypting identifiers or 'patient-identifying information') must be explored.

11 Those involved in developing health information systems should ensure that principles of best practice are incorporated during the design stage.

12 Where practicable, the internal structure and administration of databases holding patient-identifiable information should reflect the principles developed in this report.

13 The NHS number should replace the patient's name on Items-of-Service claims made by GPs as soon as is practically possible.

14 The design of new systems for transfer of prescription data should incorporate the principles developed in the Caldicott Report.

15 Future negotiations on pay and conditions for GPs should, where possible, avoid systems of payment which require patient-identifying details to be transmitted.

16 Consideration should be given to procedures for GP claims and payments which do not require patient-identifying information to be transferred, which can then be piloted.

General practitioners' workload

The Royal College of General Practitioners printed their updated information sheet on GP workload in May 2001. Its findings can be summarised as follows.

- There has been an increase in the number of part-time contracts in general practice from 5.4% in 1990 to 18.4% in 2001.

- The number of hours worked by a full-time GP when not on call has increased marginally from 38.84 to 39.21 hrs/week.

- The list size of the unrestricted principal has fallen over the last 13 years to around 1665.

- The number of consultations has fallen since 1983 from 8335 to 8030 per year in 2001.

- The number of home visits has decreased.

- The number of telephone consultations has increased marginally.

- Consultation length has increased from 8.4 to 9.36 minutes over the last 10 years.

○ (2001) How should hamsters run? Some observations about sufficient patient time in primary care. *BMJ*. **323**: 206–8.
This article summarises the fact that GPs in the UK and the USA believe they have less time for each patient, although statistically this is not the case. Doctors in fact feel stressed because there is now more that can be done, patients' expectations are higher, and there are more external forces impinging on their practice.

There is little evidence to support the view that doctors are 'running faster' in terms of both patient management and administration, despite the fact that doctors complain more.

The reasons why the workload of GPs has increased are listed below.

- The population has increased by 3%, and is now 58.4 million (the birth rate is lower, so a large proportion of this increase is due to immigration).

- Life expectancy has doubled over the last 150 years:
  - there has been a 9% increase in the geriatric population in the last decade
  - there has been a 13% increase in the population aged over 75 years in the last decade.

- The number of infant deaths has decreased.

- Divorce affects one in two marriages (social morbidity).

- Families are more spread out (i.e. there is a decreased support network).

- There are more single-parent families.

- Preventative healthcare has added 23% to the workload.

- It is now more acceptable to present with mental health problems.

- Most consultations are minor; 15% are life-threatening and need to be identified.

- Overall knowledge has increased (the *Oxford Textbook of Medicine* now runs to three volumes).

- There is increased accessibility (by telephone and email).

- GPs are accountable for practice nurse roles, etc.

- Advances in information technology.

- There are more part-time GPs.

Wanless (a former NatWest bank chief executive) has published his final report *Securing Our Future: Taking a Long-Term View* (the Wanless Report), the main points of which can be summarised as follows.

- The current method of funding healthcare, through general taxation, is fair and efficient so should not be tampered with.

- Around 70% of work currently done by doctors could be done by nurses and other healthcare professionals.

- Medical services are being forced towards greater specialisation.

Stress and burnout

Burnout is the end-stage response to excessive stress and dissatisfaction. No one is immune to stress, and you need to find a work pressure level that is constructive, not destructive. To do this, you need to be self-aware and recognise how stress affects you. How you then manage it will depend on whether you think the level of stress is a good thing or a bad thing. It should be actively managed with your own personal survival plan to prevent burnout in the long term.

There are four levels of human functioning – emotional, mental, behavioural and psychological.

Stress is also a physiological response to an inappropriate level of pressure. Noradrenaline levels increase and this, via the medulla, increases adrenaline production. This in turn increases ACTH levels and thus steroid production, which we all know improves your immunity and ability to deal with stress. When you stop working or go on holiday, all of this falls apart and you develop a cold!

People who are heading towards burnout go through four stages – overwork, frustration, resentment and finally depression (with burnout). It has always been acceptable to complain about stress, but it has not been acceptable to have symptoms, as these are interpreted as a sign of weakness. As GPs we need to be aware of the well-being of our employees and ourselves.

Causes of stress

These include the following:

- escalating workload
- frequently imposed change
- patients' expectations
- fear of litigation
- conflict (e.g. between career and family life)
- lack of career structure, etc.

Predisposing factors

In the doctor, these include the following:

- type A personality, obsessional personality
- conscientiousness, high personal standards
- reluctance to decline work
- reluctance to delegate
- competitive nature
- fear of failure to match colleagues' achievements.

In the practice, they include the following:

- single-handed or dysfunctional partnership
- professional isolation
- repeated interruptions
- unpredictable work
- long hours, out-of-hours cover
- lack of variety, no challenge
- lack of peer recognition.

In society, predisposing factors include the following:

- increase in patients' expectations
- shift of work from secondary care
- increasing litigation and complaints
- imposed change and political agendas.

Signs to look for include the following:

- poor time keeping and decision making
- sick leave
- increasing frequency of mistakes
- strained relationships.

What can we do for our employees?

- Understand that inappropriate pressures lead to stress; differentiate between pressure and stress.
- Conduct staff appraisals/make personal development plans.
- Hold practice development sessions:
  - review attitudes to stress
  - audit – establish a baseline, make the issue less confrontational, measure the effectiveness of any strategy
  - develop skills in dealing with pressure – assertiveness (not aggression) and increased resilience – by creating a balance and developing your own strategy for dealing with pressure.
- Be vigilant; observe individuals.

- Develop your own helping skills.

○ (1993) What can we do to avoid burnout ourselves? *Br J Gen Pract.*
  This article made the following recommendations.
  - Give trainees realistic expectations of general practice.
  - Choose the right job.
  - Develop practice support systems as well as personal ones (e.g. groups outside work).
  - Be assertive.
  - Develop time-management skills.
  - Be aware of your own response to stress.

Other considerations

Delegate, prioritise, keep up to date, audit, develop practice policies, balance your life (maintain outside interests), and make sure that you have a plan for dealing with stress. Organise your workload with realistic targets. Also take time out for exercise and for other hobbies (i.e. strike a balance in your professional/personal life).

How you manage pressure, stress or burnout is up to you, but make sure that you do manage it, otherwise someone will take it in hand and you will be 'managed' as someone else deems appropriate – not a comfortable situation.

The difficult patient

This is an inevitable problem for us all, and it happens for different reasons (doctor, patient and/or external factors). Heartsink patients represent a different group of people to frequent attenders.

As early as 1951, Groves defined four types of difficult patient:

1 *Dependent clinger* – grateful, but seeking reassurance for minor ailments

2 *Entitled demander* – complains about imagined shortcomings in the service provided

3 *Manipulative health rejector* – has symptoms that the doctor cannot improve

4 *Self-destructive denier* – refuses to accept that their behaviour affects their illness, and will not modify their habits.

○ Groves (1978) *NEJM.* **298**: 883–7.
  Groves defines heartsinks as patients who most physicians would dread having to treat – those who engender negative feelings.

Heartsink patients are often over-investigated or referred unnecessarily, particularly if they are seeing several GPs and no one doctor takes responsibility for the patient. It is important for your own sanity (as well as being in the patient's best interest) to develop coping strategies and a sensible, thorough approach to the heartsink patient.

Coping strategies

- Recognise your own feelings.

- Accept that heartsinks will occur.

- Review the patient's notes.

- Set goal limits.

- Assume ownership of a problem and review it regularly.

- Set limits for the patient.

- Challenge inappropriate demands.

- Hold peer group meetings/Balint groups.

- Consider alternative sources of therapy.

○ Mathers (1995) *Br J Gen Pract*.
   Mathers looked at the heartsink patient's GPs and found that doctors who had a low level of job satisfaction and no postgraduate qualifications reported more heartsink patients. It is important to recognise this association – for our own self-preservation. If we are stressed, our coping mechanisms begin to fail and we start heading towards burnout.

Chronic disease management

Chronic diseases are the main cause of morbidity and mortality in developed countries (having overtaken infectious diseases), and they account for almost a quarter of GPs' workload according to recent statistics.

A relatively recent issue of the *British Medical Journal* (26 October 2001) was dedicated to managing chronic diseases (following the success of similar theme issues in previous years).

○ (2001) *BMJ*. **323**: 945–6.
   This editorial reiterated the fact that the best outcomes depend upon competent self-management and decision making by patients, as well as clinical treatments. It also highlights the frequent co-occurence of mental disorders.

The elements of a chronic disease management programme include the following:

- clinical guidelines

- patient-friendly information which is accessible

- continuous quality improvement and clinical audit

- access to specialist care

- resource management techniques and systems

- case management

- patient education and counselling
- tracking systems
- national disease registers.

Having chronic disease morbidity registers allows the audit of standards such as compliance and prescribing. This in turn enables better planning of services and necessary changes. The data that are extracted are dependent on the accuracy of diagnosis and coding.

Further issues

- Care must be organised. If a system is methodical, it reduces the risk of error. The use of computers is very helpful both in terms of speed (once the data are input) and for audit when trying to improve quality. Protocols need to be in place, but should be flexible enough to suit the patient.

- The patient should be the most important member of the team. It is their life, and in essence we are there in an advisory capacity.

- Ethical issues arise when giving the patient the diagnosis of a chronic disease and then motivating them with regard to management and compliance, when they consider that they have been a 'normal healthy adult' until now.

- Economic and political issues arise in funding screening programmes and chronic disease clinics in an evidence-based way (medical care, equipment, administration, audit).

- No doctor or other member of the primary healthcare team should make the mistake of underestimating the psychological impact that a chronic disease can have on a person's life. It should not be trivialised, but wherever possible we should endeavour to help the patient to keep things in perspective.

The Expert Patient: A New Approach to Chronic Disease Management in the 21st Century, published in 2001, proposes that by 2004 every primary care group will have set up a lay-led training course in self-management of chronic diseases for patients. A total of £2 million is being invested in the pilot schemes.

Although all patients have needs specific to their particular disease, they also have a core of common requirements:

- knowing how to recognise and act upon symptoms
- dealing with acute attacks or exacerbations of the disease
- making the most effective use of medicines and treatment
- understanding the implications of professional advice
- establishing a stable pattern of sleep and rest, and dealing with fatigue

- accessing social and other services

- managing work and the resources of employment services

- accessing chosen leisure activities

- developing strategies to deal with the psychological consequences of illness

- learning to cope with other people's response to their chronic illness.

○ (2002) Systematic review of involving patients in the planning and development of health care. *BMJ.* **325**: 1263–5.
This review describes how involving patients has contributed to changes in the provision of services. There is not yet an evidence base looking at quality of care and satisfaction.

○ (2002) Interventions used in disease management programmes for patients with chronic illness: which one works? Meta-analysis of published reports. *BMJ.* **325**: 925–8.
There has been increasing use of disease management programmes as a means of improving the quality and efficiency of care for patients with chronic illness. This study found that many different interventions were associated with improvements in both provider adherence to guidelines and patient disease control. These included provider and patient information, patient reminders and patient financial incentives.

Guidelines

These are defined as 'systematically developed statements to assist practitioner and patient decisions about appropriate healthcare for specific clinical circumstances'.
    The aims of producing guidelines are as follows:

- to assist decision making

- to improve quality of care, effectiveness and outcome

- to standardise medical practice.

Guidelines need to be produced in an evidence-based way that acknowledges limitations such as resources, staffing and the local population for whom the guidelines are intended.
    A series of clinical articles on the various aspects of clinical guidelines was published relatively recently.

○ Woolf SH, Grol R and Hutchinson A (1999) Clinical guidelines: potential benefits, limitations and harms of clinical guidelines. *BMJ.* **318**: 527–30.

○ Shekelle PG, Woolf SH and Eccles M (1999) Clinical guidelines: developing guidelines. *BMJ.* **318**: 593–6.

○ Hurwitz B (1999) Legal and political considerations of clinical guidelines. *BMJ.* **318**: 661–4.

○ Feder G, Eccles M and Grol R (1999) Clinical guidelines: using clinical guidelines. *BMJ.* **318**: 728–30.

Guidelines in practice

Are they useful?

- Are they relevant in a clinical context?
- Are they user friendly?
- Are they evidence based?

Appraisal of guidelines takes place through the NHS Appraisal Centre for Clinical Guidelines prior to implementation.

Implementation

- The people who will be using the guidelines should have a sense of ownership, and should preferably be involved in the development (if not, then they should be involved in auditing and making amendments at a later stage).
- Local facilitators should help with this process.

Legal implications

- Guidelines can be used in court by an expert witness (but not in place of the latter) to demonstrate standards of care.
- Non-compliance to clinical guidelines does not mean that care is sub-standard.

Compliance

It can be difficult to comply with guidelines as they are not written for individual patients, but rather they reflect a consensus opinion based on the current evidence without taking into account uncertainties and ethical or cultural issues which may arise.

Potential benefits of guidelines

Benefits for patients include the following:

- improved consistency of care
- empowerment to make informed choices.

Benefits for healthcare professionals include the following:

- improved quality of clinical decisions (although to a variable degree)
- they are evidence based, so improve knowledge, highlight gaps and through audit improve quality of care.

Benefits for healthcare systems include the following:

- efficient use of resources

- distributive justice (i.e. ethical issues relating to rationing)

- improved public perception of equality.

Potential drawbacks of guidelines

- They may be incorrect/flawed/biased or conflict with other professional groups.

- They can be time-consuming to implement.

- They are written for populations, not individuals.

- They will increase the amount of resources needed (e.g. statins in cardiovascular disease).

- They need regular review.

- They do not address the complexity and uncertainties of medical practice.

Patient groups directives

These are written instructions for the supply and administration of medicines by professionals other than doctors (e.g. pharmacists, nurses, health visitors).

Their development followed changes to the Medicines Act in 2000, the overall aim being to improve patient care. They are a recognised necessity due to the advances in nurse prescribing. However, many practices do not have them in place. The process of drawing up a patient group directive can be time-consuming, and must be well thought out and involve a multidisciplinary team. For example, pharmacists who will be issuing emergency contraception not only must be competent in assessing need and explaining related issues, but also require a means of effective reimbursement for the cost of the drug.

The patient group directive needs to be detailed, and once it has been written it must be reviewed by at least one professional advisory group prior to circulation to practices.

Like any published document, it should be dated and have a plan for review.

Each direction must contain:

- the name of the business to which it applies

- the date it comes into force and is due to expire

- a description of the medicines to which it applies

- the class of health professional who may supply or administer the medicine

- signature of the doctor, dentist or pharmacist and appropriate health organisation.

- the clinical condition to which it applies

- patients to be excluded

- when further advice should be sought and more ...

Screening

Wilson's criteria (1966) can be summarised as follows.

1 The condition must be:
    - common
    - important
    - diagnosable by acceptable methods.

2 There should be a latent period during which effective interventional treatment is possible.

3 Screening must be:
    - cheap/cost-effective
    - continuous
    - safe
    - repeatable
    - non-invasive
    - acceptable to patients
    - such that the test has a high positive predictive value.

4 Treatment must be available.

Technically, screening is a form of secondary prevention (i.e. it involves identifying presymptomatic disease before significant damage is done).

Examples of primary prevention would include immunisation, water sanitation, etc. Tertiary prevention is about limiting complications (e.g. in diabetic care).

When establishing a screening programme you need to consider the ethics. Increasing numbers of studies are looking at the negative effects of screening. For example, a normal cholesterol result may mean that a patient's diet subsequently lapses because they feel justified in indulging more often. Another example would be the psychological implications of being given a positive result after, say, chlamydia screening.

○ (1999) *BMJ*.
Because of the implications mentioned above, this editorial discussed the issues relating to obtaining consent, emphasising the importance of shared decision making and the patient's autonomy.

Medicine and the Internet

It is accepted that the Internet can improve communication and access both among professionals and with patients.

○ (1999) *BMJ*. **319**: 1294–6.
   An estimated 25 million people use the Internet to access health information, of whom 27% are female and 15% are male.

One of the biggest problems with information on the Internet is that there is no quality control/regulation (i.e. there is no guarantee that the information is reliable), which means that as GPs we may need to guide our patients. Health on the Net (www.hon.ch/) is an international organisation which provides a database of evaluated health material. Any website health information which displays the HON logo was developed in accordance with this foundation's guidelines.

NHSnet

As part of the Government directive, all GP practices should be connected to NHSnet. It is planned that health records will be networked, thus allowing doctors 24-hour access. Inevitably this raises data protection issues, which are addressed in the Caldicott Report 1999. Appointments as well as X-ray and pathology requests will be made online, and pharmacists will accept prescriptions electronically.

   The potential applications of NHSnet are limited only by us. At whatever speed changes are implemented, the systems that are used need to have been thought through in terms of confidentiality (patient and doctor), data protection and litigation issues. They also need to be quick and user-friendly.

European Computer Driving License (ECDL) Programme

This is a scheme to allow all NHS staff to train online and be examined to ECDL standards, over seven modules of basic skills.

   The scheme was developed in Finland in 1988, and 200 000 people in the UK are now registered.

   More information is available at www.nhsia.nhs.uk.

Evidenced-based medicine

Evidenced-based medicine (EBM) was coined as a buzz phrase in the early 1990s, and has increased our awareness of research studies and improved our knowledge base within the profession as a whole. This can give our patients the confidence that we are up to date and giving them appropriate advice.

   Research findings ('the evidence') are almost never black and white, and often only look at a specific point at the expense of other issues (e.g. resources). This leaves us the clinicians (who are not the best at interpreting studies) with the dilemma of how – or indeed if – we should use certain findings.

○ (2001) Why GPs do not implement evidence: qualitative study. *BMJ*. **323**: 1100–2.
   This article pointed out that GPs are generally cautious about the evidence-based model. They are reluctant to jeopardise relationships with patients, and patients are often unwilling to take certain drugs. It concluded that GPs regarded clinical evidence as a square peg to be fitted in the round hole of a patient's life. The process of implementation is complex, fluid and adaptive.

Sources of evidence are diverse, but the gold standard is held to be a meta-analysis of randomised controlled trials. The Cochrane Reviews are one point at which to access some such information, although their validity has recently been questioned.

○ (2001) Quality of Cochrane Reviews: assessment of sample from 1998. *BMJ*. **323**: 829-32.
This review concluded that although the Cochrane database is a key source of evidence, users should interpret reviews cautiously, especially if experimental interventions are advocated. In nine out of 53 reviews it was found that the evidence did not support the conclusions.

The Cochrane Collaboration has taken steps to improve the quality of its reviews following the highlighting of minor problems by this study.

DARE (Database of Abstracts of Reviews) is another tool forming part of the Cochrane Library which contains systematic reviews. This can be accessed free of charge at www.nhscrd.york.ac.uk.

Alternatively, you can telephone 01904 433707 and someone will perform the search for you.

○ (2002) *Effectiveness Matters.* **6**(2) gives an overview of DARE.

○ (2003) Validation of the Fresno test of competence in evidence-based medicine. *BMJ*. **236**: 319–21.
This test has been developed by the Fresno Medical Education Program in California. It is a tool for assessing knowledge and skill (ability) in teaching evidence-based medicine, and can identify the strengths and weaknesses of curricula and individuals. It has a standardised grading system and seems to be valid, although the authors point out that familiarity may have led to unrealistic scoring.

Death certification

Death certification provides legal evidence of the fact and cause(s) of death, which then allows the death to be registered. It is important to be as accurate as possible – a mode of dying is not acceptable.

Terms which imply a mode of dying include the following:

- asphyxia
- asthenia
- brain failure
- cachexia
- cardiac arrest
- cardiac failure
- coma
- debility
- exhaustion
- hepatic failure
- renal failure

- respiratory arrest
- shock
- syncope
- Uraemia
- vagal inhibition.

Old age can only be cited as a cause of death if the person is over 70 years of age and a more specific cause of death cannot be given.

Duties of the medical practitioner of the deceased include the following.

- If you were in attendance in the deceased's last illness, you are required to certify the cause of death.
- You are legally responsible for the delivery of the death certificate to the registrar. This may be done in person, by post or by a relative (or other person).
- You should also complete the notice to informant (attached to the death certificate) and the counterfoil in the book for your records.

There are three types of certificate:

- Medical Certificate of cause of death (Form 66) – for any death after the first 28 days of life
- Neonatal Death Certificate (Form 65) – for any live-born death within 28 days of birth
- Certificate of Stillbirth (Form 34) – for any death of an infant after 34 weeks of pregnancy which showed no signs of life after delivery from the mother.

When to refer to the coroner

There is no statutory duty to report to the coroner (this would otherwise be done by the registrar), but voluntary reporting where suggested avoids unnecessary delay and anxiety for the relatives.

A death should be referred if:

- the cause of death is unknown
- the deceased has not been seen by the certifying doctor either after death or within 14 days before death
- the death was violent, unnatural or suspicious
- the death may be due to an accident (whenever it occurred)
- the death may be due to self-neglect or neglect by others
- the death may be due to industrial disease or related to the deceased's employment

- the death may be due to an abortion

- the death occurred during an operation or before recovery from the effects of an anaesthetic

- the death may be suicide

- The death occured during, or shortly after, detention in police or prison custody.

Advance directives ('living wills')

In medieval times a good death was a prepared death. Advance directives are statements (usually written and formally witnessed) made by a person about the medical care that they do and do not want if they become incompetent in the future.

○ (2001) Is there such a thing as a life not worth living? *BMJ*. **322**: 1481–3.
This article debates the practical difficulties of measurement and the ethical issues associated with determining quality of life in situations where a life has been judged to have no quality. Patients who are dying may find some quality in life even when the latter is assessed by current measures as abysmal. The use of proxies is touched upon as a problem for similar reasons, namely the disparity between an observer's assessment and the patient's own evaluation.

○ (2001) *BMJ*. **323**: 1079–80.
This editorial was written in the light of the Diane Pretty test case. 'If death is in a patient's best interest, then death constitutes a moral good.'

Legally the whole subject of advance directives is complicated. At present there are six types of advance statement:

1 a requesting statement reflecting an individual's aspirations and preferences

2 a statement of general beliefs and aspects of life that the individual values

3 a statement naming a proxy

4 a directive giving clear instructions that relate to some or all of treatment

5 a statement specifying a degree of irreversible deterioration after which no life-sustaining treatment should be given

6 a combination of all of the above.

An advance directive should not preclude the provision of basic care defined as maintenance of bodily cleanliness, relief of sustained pain, and provision of *oral* nutrition and hydration.

The current legal situation in the UK

- The patient must be competent at the time of declaration.

- He or she must be informed in broad terms about the nature and effect of treatments and procedures.

- He or she must have anticipated and intended the declaration to apply to the circumstances that subsequently arise.

- He or she must be free from undue influence when issuing the declaration.

○ (1998) Advance directives in the UK: legal, ethical and practical considerations. *BMJ*. **48**: 1263–6.
   This paper highlights the fact that most articles written on the subject cover legal or practical matters, and it points out that it is not in the best interest of the doctor or the patient to reduce medical ethics to medical law.

A GP is likely to be involved with advance directives in one of two ways:

1 when advising patients when advance directives may be appropriate, and the phrasing of the directive

2 as a repository of the advance directive, which would be forwarded to the appropriate department on request.

An advance directive has been legally binding on a doctor in common law since 1994, and has been endorsed by the British Medical Association since 1995, and by the legal profession. Euthanasia is illegal in the UK, and a World Medical Association resolution has condemned it as unethical. Most experts believe that directives should be reviewed periodically (e.g. every 5 years).

Formatted versions are available from either the Terence Higgins Trust (0171 831 0330) or the Voluntary Euthanasia Society (0171 937 7770).

Medic Alert are allowed to engrave bracelets advising that the patient has a living will. They can keep a copy and fax it to the appropriate department or read it to the paramedics.

○ General Medical Council (2002) *Withholding and Withdrawing Life-Prolonging Treatments. Good practice in decision making*. General Medical Council, London; www.gmc-uk.org
   This publication looks at guiding principles and our ethical obligations to show respect for human life, the dilemmas of starting and stopping treatment, a framework of good practice, and areas of special consideration.

○ (2003) Assisted suicide and euthanasia in Switzerland: allowing a role for non-physicians. *BMJ*. **326**: 271–3.
   This is an educational publication. Assisted suicide is not a criminal act under Swiss law, and a physician's professional ethics could lead to a personal conflict about assisting death. Altruistic assisted suicide by non-physicians is legal in Switzerland, which has enabled certain issues to be separated, but the whole debate will certainly continue.

Integrated/alternative medicine

Complementary medicine (which focuses on health and healing) and conventional medicine (which focuses on disease and treatment) have traditionally been distinct from one another, but recently they have become increasingly integrated. This means that complementary medicine will have to be subject to similar clinical, scientific and regulatory standards to those that are applied to conventional health-care.

○ (1999) *BMJ*. **319**: 901–4.
   It is estimated that 30% of the UK population use alternative medicines and currently 40% of GPs in the UK offer access to complementary treatment.

Public awareness and use of complementary medicine have increased dramatically over the last 10 years, but many complementary practitioners remain unregulated, although osteopaths and chiropractors are now becoming the exception here.

○ (2001) Regulation in complementary and alternative medicine. *BMJ*. **322**: 158–60.
   This article looks at regulation in terms of accountability, conduct, ongoing education and the prospects for various disciplines following the recommendations made by the House of Lords Select Committee on Science and Technology. Provision of complementary medicine on the NHS might protect patients from unqualified practitioners, and ensure minimum standards and proper regulation.

○ (2001) *Ann Intern Med*. **135**: 344–51.
   A total of 831 people in the USA who use alternative/complementary medicine were surveyed.
   • Around 80% thought that the combination of complementary and conventional medicine was superior to either alone.
   • Most saw a conventional doctor first.
   • Around 70% did not subsequently disclose that they were seeing a complementary therapist, because this was not thought to be any of the doctor's business, rather than this information being withheld for fear of criticism.

○ (2001) *Br J Gen Pract*. **51**: 914–16.
   This cross-sectional survey of 904 parents looked at repeated use of complementary medicine in children. It was found that 17.9% had used complementary treatments for their children.

Acupuncture

On the basis of current evidence, acupuncture is effective in treating nausea and vomiting, back pain, dental pain and migraine. The incidence of adverse reactions to acupuncture is relatively low. It is the most popular form of complementary therapy among GPs (used by 47%). This popularity has only emerged in the UK over the last 20 years, although the technique has been used for many thousands of years in Chinese medicine.

Non-medical acupuncturists should be members of the British Acupuncture Council, which has strict educational criteria and a code of practice. Physiotherapists may belong to the Acupuncture Association of Chartered Physiotherapists.

○ (2001) Adverse events following acupuncture: prospective survey of 32 000 consultations with doctors and physiotherapists. *BMJ*. **323**: 485–6 (there is an accompanying editorial).
   This study found that no adverse events were reported after 34 407 acupuncture treatments from data collected over a 4-week period. It did not look at patients' experiences of adverse events, but is nevertheless encouraging/reassuring research.

Herbal remedies

Again popularity in the UK means that sales are increasing by 20% a year. The users of these remedies often have the belief that 'herbal equals natural', and that it is both safe and cheaper than conventional medicine, with no side-effects. However, many herbal products do have side-effects and can interact with other drugs.

As there is little legislation for control, doses of preparations can vary widely, even in the same product. Some products may also contain conventional medicines (e.g. one eczema cream was recently found to contain high doses of dexamethasone, although it had been advertised as a natural product).

- *Ginseng*: This is teratogenic, increases the international normalised ratio (INR) and may also increase blood pressure, and interacts with digoxin. There are several varieties. The active ingredients (ginsenosides) are antioxidants and enhance nitrate production.

- *St John's Wort*: (*see* section on depression, pages 31–5). This is a weak SSRI and antiviral drug. It is a liver-enzyme inducer, so may reduce the concentrations of digoxin, carbamazepine, warfarin and the oral contraceptive pill. It also interacts with several other drugs.

- *Ginkgo biloba*: (*see* section on dementia, pages 46–9). This is used to delay clinical progression of dementia. It is a potent inhibitor of platelet-activating factor, so can increase the risk of bleeds (including intracerebral bleeding) in patients on aspirin or warfarin.

The herbal advice line is staffed by members of the National Institute of Medical Herbalists. They can give advice on remedies, interactions, and use of herbal products in children and during pregnancy. The line is open Monday to Friday, 9a.m.–1p.m. Tel: 0906 802 0117.

Homeopathy

This needs to be distinguished from herbal remedies. Homeopathic remedies contain minute or non-existent amounts of the original substance, and are prepared by successive dilutions.

Although to our knowledge there are insufficient randomised controlled trials to advocate the use of homeopathic treatments in specific conditions, many people report having benefited from them.

○ (1997) *Lancet*. **350**: 834–43.
  This meta-analysis of 100 randomised controlled trials concluded that their results were not compatible with the hypothesis that the clinical effects of homeopathy were completely due to the placebo effect. Researchers at York University found that there was not enough evidence to support homeopathy as a treatment for any specific conditions.

Homeopathy – A Guide for GPs (from the Faculty of Homeopathy) describes a range of NHS services that are now available, and gives details of how GPs can refer patients.

Glasgow and London Homeopathic Hospitals are the two leading bodies in research in this field, but funding is severely lacking, more so than in other areas of medicine.

The Faculty of Homeopathy Website (www.trusthomeopathy.org/faculty) is a good source of information.

Antioxidants

These include ginseng, β-carotene, vitamins C and E, minerals such as zinc and copper, flavonoids, etc.

Most of the available evidence is in the form of cohort studies. As yet there seems to be insufficient evidence that taking antioxidants offers much in the way of benefit to healthy people.

Air travel

When booking our holidays and long-haul flights, few of us will give much thought to our health, but increasingly as GPs we will be asked questions about risk and recommendations for prevention of, for example, deep vein thrombosis (DVT).

In response to the House of Lords report on health and air travel (November 2000), the Department of Health has published advice for passengers (this can be found at www.doh.gov.uk/dvt).

The absolute risk of thrombosis is small. The longer the duration of travel, the higher the apparent risk, although there is no lower limit below which it is 'safe'. As the risks for thrombosis are additive, short sequential flights probably increase the risk. Factors that put people at risk on long-haul flights include cramped conditions, varying air pressure and oxygen concentration, and dehydration (with or without excess alcohol consumption). Certain factors put some people at higher risk than others, including heart disease, pregnancy, the pill, HRT, a family history of DVT, recent major leg surgery and increasing age.

Sensible advice is lacking in evidence, but the general consensus is as follows.

- Move around in the seat and in the cabin as much as possible.

- Rotate ankles and flex calf muscles regularly.

- Avoid alcohol and caffeine.

- Avoid dehydration (i.e. drink plenty of water).

TED stockings

Mediven travel stockings (which exert a pressure of 20 mmHg at the ankle) have been shown to reduce the incidence of DVT in travellers. There is no evidence for the effectiveness of lower compression stockings.

Aspirin

The benefits of aspirin are arterial rather than venous. To our knowledge, no published study has shown any reduction in the risk of thrombosis in travellers with aspirin use. It is important to be aware of the gastrointestinal risk and the fact that some clinics are advising taking 150 mg the day before travel.

Subcutaneous heparin

This is indicated in high-risk patients, and it does reduce the risk of DVT. Usually one injection 2–4 hours before travel is adequate. If the patient is on warfarin there is no additional benefit.

Airogym

This is an inflatable cushion that is placed under the feet which simulates walking when pressed. So far the results are encouraging, but as yet there have been no published trials.

Medical ethics

> Understanding the law helps us deal with disputes; a proper understanding of medical ethics will help us work in true partnership with our patients.
>
> (Dr Cox, 8 November 2001)

This is a source of anxiety for many, especially when approaching exams like the MRCGP oral. The General Medical Council requires that medical ethics be a core subject in the medical curriculum, and also that there should be a medical ethics curriculum. Try not to be daunted by the subject. Most of what you need you already know, but it is now a case of formulating a way of thinking and talking about ethical principles, using an ethical model that you can apply to a given situation.

Medical ethics applies to all areas of medicine, including end-of-life decisions, medical error, priority setting, biotechnology, education, consent and confidentiality.

○ (2000) Ethics and communication skills. *Medicine*. **28**.
  This provides an excellent narrative, not just on ethics.

Questions on ethical values cannot be solved by simply applying an algorithm. If we are to practise medicine in a way that we think is right, we must:

- clarify what value judgements are relevant in a specific clinical situation
- be aware of the relevant issues
- subject our views to critical analysis to ensure that they are logical and consistent
- adapt or change our views in the light of such analysis.

In addition we must practise medicine in a legal framework.
  The *four principles approach* can be summarised as follows:

- respect for *autonomy* ('self-rule') – help patients to make their own decisions and respect those decisions even if you do not agree with them
- *beneficence* (do good) – this involves doing what is best for the patient, but who is the judge of what is best? This may conflict with autonomy

- *Non-maleficence* (avoiding harm) – in most cases this does not add anything to the principle of beneficence

- *Justice* – this incorporates time and resources.

The Declaration of Helsinki (revised for the fifth time by the World Medical Association) was adopted in 1964 and sets out widely accepted ethical principles for medical research involving human subjects.

○ (2001) What are the effects of the fifth revision of the Declaration of Helsinki? *BMJ*. **323**: 1417–23.

○ (2001) Revising and implementing the Tavistock principles for everybody in health care. *BMJ*. **323**: 616–20.
The Tavistock Group published their original five principles in 1999. The principles are not evidence based, but are intended to serve as an ethical framework for those working to improve medical error.

Important ethical concepts of the Tavistock Group

- *Rights* – people have a right to health and healthcare.

- *Balance* – care of individual patients is central, but the health of the population is also our concern.

- *Comprehensiveness* – in addition to treating illness, we have an obligation to ease suffering, minimise disability, prevent disease and promote health.

- *Co-operation* – healthcare only succeeds if we co-operate with those we serve, each other and those in other sectors.

- *Improvement* – improving healthcare is a serious and continuing responsibility.

- *Safety* – do no harm.

- *Openness* – being open, honest and trustworthy is vital in healthcare.

Fraser guidelines

Confidentiality is important in all patients but young patients think that their parents can access their records and that they have to be over 16 to see a health professional without their parents. This is not the case.

A young person is competent to consent to treatment if:

- the young person understands the doctor's advice

- the doctor cannot persuade the young person to inform his or her parents or allow the doctor to inform parents that he or she is seeking contraceptive advice

- the young person is very likely to begin, or continue having, intercourse with or without contraceptive treatment

- unless he or she receives contraceptive treatment, the young person's physical or mental health, or both, are likely to suffer

- the young person's best interests require the doctor to give contraceptive advice, treatment, or both, without parental consent.

○ (2000) Access by the unaccompanied under-16-year-old adolescent to general practice without parental consent. *J Fam Plan Reprod Health*. **29**(4): 205–7.

Consultation models

The consultation – you cannot ignore it, for it is central to what we do every day.

The most likely place for specific questions to come up is in the oral, but once you are familiar with the different models, you could quote them left, right and centre. The frameworks of different models can even help with your answers to the written paper. However, in the orals the examiners must get rather tired of people reciting Neighbour and Pendleton – although well done for remembering this!

What we have tried to do in this section is give a brief summary of several models. Of course, this is no substitute for reading the original texts from cover to cover, but it is probably a little easier to digest at this stage.

It is worth noting that the formal history-taking part of clinical management, if used prematurely, can stifle the patient's agenda. The patient's initial narrative is an important part of the consultation. It has been proved, contrary to popular belief, that the majority of patients will not go on talking indefinitely, but will stop within less than 1 minute. Allowing the patient to get their problem off their chest while uninterrupted greatly increases satisfaction on all sides.

○ (2002) The consultation. *BMJ*. **324**: 1567–9.
   This is a clinical review that looks at consultation technique, provision of information and the ability to motivate changes in behaviour. It goes through aspects of the consultation and makes suggestions that could potentially improve your facilitatory skills.

○ (2002) Key communication skills and how to acquire them. *BMJ*. **325**: 697–700.
   This was another clinical review which found that doctors with good communication skills identified problems more accurately and had greater job satisfaction, and their patients were more satisfied with their care.

○ (2003) William Pickles Lecture by Jacky Hayden. *Br J Gen Pract*. **53**: 143–8.
   William Pickles was a GP in Aysgarth, and he was well respected as a patient-centred doctor. This is an interesting article on medical teaching and personal and social competence. It highlights the characteristics of a patient-centred doctor as including the following:
   - explores the disease and the effects on and expectations of the patient
   - understands the whole person
   - finds common ground in managing a problem
   - incorporates health promotion
   - is realistic about the time and resources needed.

Balint model

This is a psychological model of the doctor–patient relationship. The understanding that doctors have feelings and that these have a function within the consultation forms part of the model.

Balint explains that a patient's problem will have psychological and physical components, and that these will be interlinked. Indeed, psychological problems may manifest themselves clinically. Individual doctors vary in their awareness of these points, but they can be trained to be more sensitive and aware.

Important features of the Balint model include the following:

- the doctor as a drug
- the child of a patient may be brought with a trivial problem to enable the patient to make contact (i.e. with the child as the presenting complaint)
- elimination by appropriate examination
- collusion of anonymity.

Berne's transactional analysis

○ Berne E (1968) *Games People Play*. Penguin Books, London.

This model looks at the roles that patients and doctors play within the consultation, and identifies three 'ego' states:

- parent – critical or caring
- adult – logical
- child – dependent.

This is a useful model for analysing why consultations go wrong. Often a doctor will flit between adult and parent state, and the patient will flit between adult and child (and parent to a lesser degree). Imagine a consultation in which both the doctor and the patient assumed the role of 'child'. I am sure you would agree that it would be likely to be dysfunctional.

Stott and Davis model

This is a four-part model:

Management of presenting problem	Management of continuing problem
Modification of health-seeking behaviour	Opportunistic health promotion

This is probably the way many of us deal with a consultation, on the face of it.

Neighbour's model: the inner consultation

This is a popular 'check point model'. It consists of the following steps.

1 *Connecting* – establishing a relationship; this needs rapport-building skills.

2 *Summarising* – 'What I am hearing is …'; this needs the ability to listen and the skills to facilitate effective assessment.

3 *Hand over* – responsibility is given to the patient; this needs good communication skills to hand over the responsibility for management, as it involves negotiating and influencing (to a certain extent).

4 *Safety-netting* – 'Have I missed anything?', and instructions for follow up if …; this needs predictive skills to suggest contingency plans for the worst-case scenario.

5 *Housekeeping* – 'Am I fit for the next patient?'; this needs self-awareness and the ability to file one consultation so that there is no effect on the next.

Pendleton model

This is also known as the *social skills model*. It has seven tasks.

1 Define the reason for the patient's attendance, including the following:
   • the nature and history of the problems
   • their aetiology
   • the patient's ideas, concerns and expectations
   • the effects of the problem.
2 Consider other problems:
   • continuing other problems
   • at-risk factors.
3 Choose with the patient an appropriate action for each problem.

4 Achieve a shared understanding of the problems with the patient.

5 Involve the patient in the management of their case, and involve them in acceptance of appropriate responsibility for it.

6 Use time and resources appropriately.

7 Establish or maintain a relationship with the patient which helps in the achievement of other tasks.

Byrne and Long model

This is a six-point 'time-sequence model' (i.e. it is based on the observed sequence of events).

1 The doctor establishes a relationship with the patient.

2 The doctor attempts to discover the patient's reason for attendance.

3 The doctor conducts a verbal (and physical) examination.

4 The doctor (with or without the patient) considers the problems.

5 The doctor (with or without the patient) makes a further plan (e.g. investigation, treatment, etc.).

6 The consultation is terminated, usually by the doctor.

Middleton agenda model

This is a four-point dynamic model in which the patient's agenda is paramount. It is not task orientated.

1 *Patient's agenda* – this includes the ideas and reasoning which underlie the problems presented.

2 *Doctor's agenda* – this includes risk factors, continuing problems, public health agenda, partnerships and personal agendas.

3 *Communication skills* – these can be chosen to reconcile the agendas (e.g. facilitation and negotiation).

4 *Negotiated plan* – this includes management of problems and health promotion.

Triaxial model

This model looks at the patient's problems in physical, psychological and social terms.

Heron model

This is a six-category intervention model (i.e. the doctor can use any of six types of intervention).

1 *Prescriptive* – instructions given.

2 *Informative* – explanations given.

3 *Confronting* – challenging but caring (e.g. on behaviour/presentation).

4 *Cathartic* – aids release of emotions (e.g. anger, laughter, tears).

5 *Catalytic* – encourages patient's exploration of their feelings, thoughts and behaviour.

6 *Supportive* – of the problems and solutions presented.

Calgary–Cambridge guide

This can be summarised as follows.

1 *Initiating the session*:
   - establishing a rapport
   - identifying reasons for the consultation.

2 *Gathering information*:
   - exploration of the problem
   - understanding the patient's perspective
   - providing structure for the consultation.

3 *Building the relationship*:
   - providing the correct amount and type of information
   - aiding accurate recall and understanding
   - achieving a shared understanding
   - shared decision making
   - negotiating a management plan.

4 *Closing the session*:
   - final summary.

5 *Contracting* – establish a plan/contract with the patient.

6 *Safety-netting* – similar to Neighbour's model.

7 *Final check* – before moving on.

Critical reading

At the risk of sounding like a secondary-school teacher, your ability to assess the quality of the work that has been published will only improve if you practise. If you decide to take the MRCGP, usually three of the questions in the written paper are on critical appraisal. These seem to take more time to answer than candidates often appreciate. This brings us back to the issue of practice.

It is useful to have a simple critical appraisal template that you can apply in order to structure the way in which you read and then apply your answers. We have provided some examples of different methods you can try.

Reader

○ (1994) *Br J Gen Pract.* **44**: 83–5.

R   Relevance:
   - to general practice
   - to your environment
   - general awareness.
E   Education:
   - behaviour modification
   - challenges to practices and beliefs.

A   Applicability:
- to own environment
- generalisability.
D   Discrimination:
- quality of the study
- type of study: descriptive/randomised controlled trial
- sample size
- selection
- controls
- bias
- results
- statistics
- conclusions.
E   Evaluation:
- reflection.
R   Reaction:
- implementation.

Remember always to try and be positive about a study first.

Template for critical appraisal

1 *Summary*
- Concise statement of topic and conclusions.

2 *Introduction*
- Is there a clear outline?

3 *Methods and design*
- Are the selection and sample size appropriate?
- What are the strengths and limitations?

4 *Results*
- Is presentation clear?
- Are results both clinically and statistically significant?

5 *Discussion*
- Are statements true?

Keele University model

This method will help you to obtain the important information from each section (i.e. summarise the paper). This provides the basis for evaluating it.

1 *Is it of interest?*
- Look at the abstract, title, authors etc.

2 *Motivation: why was it done?*
   - Introduction? Is it clear?
   - Who funded the research?

3 *Design: how was it done?*
   - Look at the methods: sample, recruitment, numbers, collection of data.
   - Measurements: are they valid/reliable?
   - Analysis: what statistics were used?
   - Any ethical problems or bias?

4 *Results: what did it find?*
   - Look at the results: are the data described and do the numbers add up?
   - Was statistical significance assessed?
   - Were all of the data used?

5 *Conclusions: what are the implications?*
   - Look at the discussion.
   - Has anything been overlooked?
   - Are the findings relevant?

6 *Is there anything else of interest?*
   - For example, references.

Appraisal

1 Is the hypothesis clearly described?
2 Are the outcomes measured clearly described? If these are first mentioned in the results section, then the answer to this is no.
3 Are the characteristics of groups (e.g. inclusion/exclusion criteria) clearly described?
4 Are the interventions clearly described?
5 Are the main findings clearly described?
6 Does the study provide estimates of random variability in the data for the main outcomes?
   - If the data are non-normally distributed, the interquartile range should be quoted.
   - If the data has a normal distribution, the standard error of the mean, standard deviation and confidence intervals should be used.
7 Have important adverse events been reported?
8 Have the characteristics of patients who were lost to follow-up been reported?
9 Have actual probability values been reported (e.g. $P = 0.04$ rather than $P < 0.05$)?

External validity

10 Were the subjects representative of the population?
11 Were the staff and facilities representative of the treatment that the majority of patients would receive?

Internal validity and bias (think selection and information)

12 Was the study blinded?
13 Were the statistical tests used appropriate?
  • Non-parametric tests should be used for data that are not normally distributed.
14 Was compliance with the intervention reliable?
15 Were the main outcome measurements that were used reliable?

Implications of the study (the final part of appraisal)

1 What is its general importance in the light of other research?

2 Can you extrapolate from the study group to general practice?

3 Is the size of the observed result important? The answer to this question may be no, even if the results are statistically significant.

4 If you conclude that the results are important, what are their implications?
  • For patients?
  • For GPs?
    – workload
    – financial implications
    – education
    – resources
    – other members of the primary healthcare team.
  • For wider issues: ethics, right to choose.

Qualitative research

The approach is similar to that for quantitative appraisal.

• Focus on methods (e.g. interview techniques and settings) (source of internal bias), as well as the role of the researcher and their qualifications.

• Look at the quality-control measures used (e.g. content analysis, grounded theory).

• In qualitative research, the conclusions and discussion are not separate.

Statistics

Statistics is about gathering, communicating, analysing and interpreting information. In medical research we tend to use *inferential statistics,* in that we reach conclusions about a sample that has been drawn from the population.

When critiquing papers, or embarking on research or audit yourself, you need to have a fundamental understanding of the basics. I shall attempt to put this in simple terms and explain things which may otherwise appear to be double Dutch.

There are two distinct types of data.

1 *Qualitative data* – descriptive information.

2 *Quantitative data* – numerical information.

Quantitative data can be either *continuous* (e.g. 0.1 kg to 44 kg, all values within the span are possible) or they can be *discrete*, usually obtained by counting (e.g. 0, 1, 2, 3 ... , such as the number of moles present or shoe size).

Bar charts

A bar chart is a graphical representation of values/numbers.

- The height of each column is proportional to the frequency that it represents.
- Each column should have the same width.

An example of a bar chart is shown below.
   There is obviously too much information lacking in this bar chart for it to be useful!

Pie chart/pie diagram

This is a circle divided into sectors at angles which are proportional to the frequency of the data that they represent.
   An example of a pie chart is shown on page 193.

Measures of location

Mode

This is the MOst commonly occurring value. It assumes that the modal class is divided into the same ratio.

Time taken to critique a paper (minutes)	Number of people
0–9.9	4
10–19.9	7
20–29.9	9
30–39.9	6
40–49.9	5
50–59.9	3
60–120	9

The mode is time 20–29.9 minutes, *not* 60–120 minutes, as this modal class is longer.
   It is possible to have more than one modal class.

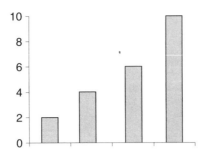

The number of packets of gum consumed per month

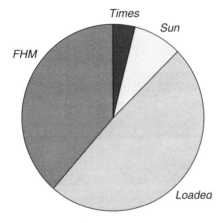

The number of times violence appeared in print

Median

This is the middle value of data once they have been placed in numerical order.

For example: 3 4 5 6 7 **7** 8 8 8 10 15

The 7 in bold typeface is the median.

Or: 0 1 2 4 5 5 6 7

The median is halfway between 4 and 5, so is 4.5.

Mean

This generally means the average.

$$\text{Mean} = \frac{\text{sum of the values}}{\text{number of values}}$$

The mean and median are a measure of symmetry or lack of it.

In a normal (Gaussian) distribution, the mode, median and mean all have the same value.

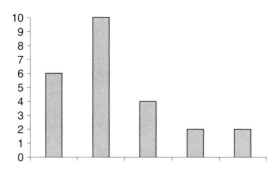

Positive skew

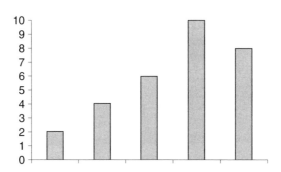

Negative skew

Measure of dispersion

Range

This is the difference between extremes (i.e. the largest and the smallest). It does not take into account anything about the distribution of the data.

Quartile spread

- The median is halfway through the data.
- The point halfway between the lower extreme and the median is the *lower quartile*.
- The point halfway between the median and the upper extreme is the *upper quartile*.
- The difference between the upper and lower quartiles is the *interquartile range*.

Standard deviation

- Whereas range and interquartile range relate to the median, standard deviation relates to the spread about the mean.

- The standard deviation uses all values, and is therefore sensitive to outliers (i.e. extreme values).

SD = square root of the variance.

$$\text{Variance} = \frac{\text{sum of the square deviations from the mean}}{n}.$$

In a normal distribution:

- 65% of values lie within 1 SD

- 95% of values lie within 2 SD

- 99% of values lie within 3 SD.

Probability

This indicates the degree of likelihood of an event happening, or the uncertainty of an event occurring.

$$\text{Probability of an outcome} = \frac{\text{number of events in the outcome}}{\text{total number of possible events}}.$$

For example, the probability of rolling a 6 when throwing a dice is 1/6.
The probability of throwing a 6 followed by another 6 is 1/6 x 1/6 = 1/36 (i.e. probability of a and b, so multiply).

The probability of throwing a 6 or a 4 is 1/6 + 1/6 = 2/6 = 1/3 (i.e. probability of a or b so add).

Errors

There are two types of error.

1 In *random error*, the sample mean deviates from the true mean despite the sample being representative.

2 In *systematic error*, the sample is not representative (i.e. there is bias).

Hypothesis test and **P-value**

This is a test of significance.

1 The first step is the statement of the null hypothesis:
   'there is no difference between the two groups under study'
   (i.e. postulate that the intervention will have no effect).

2 The second step is to conduct a test of statistical significance based on the null hypothesis:
   - t-test
   - Chi-squared test.

3 The third step is the production of a P-value from the statistical tests.

The P-value is the probability of the result occurring by chance if the null hypothesis was true.

If the P-value is small, then it is unlikely to have occurred by chance (i.e. it is a significant result). Usually $P < 0.05$ indicates a significant result.

If $P < 0.01$, the result is highly significant (i.e. it is likely to have occurred by chance in less than 1% of cases).

Note that P-values are irrelevant in the following circumstances:

- poor design of trial

- bias

- trial affected by confounding factors.

Therefore it is important to appraise the study first.

If there is a small sample size, then you will be unable to detect a statistically significant difference when there may be one. This is referred to as the power of the study.

Confidence intervals

Confidence intervals (CI) are another way of assessing the effects of chance (c.f. P-value). They are a way of communicating the level of uncertainty, and they can be calculated for various statistical analyses (e.g. odds ratios, relative risks, risk difference, sensitivity, specificity, etc.).

- There is an upper and a lower value and, assuming that the study was not biased, the true value can be expected to lie between these two values.

- Most studies use 95% CI or 95% confidence limits. This is usually two standard deviations either side of the mean.

- The wider the range of CI, the less certain/significant the results are. The more people there are in the study, the smaller the interval will be.

- If the CI range includes zero, the result is not statistically significant.

- If the results are expressed as a ratio, then a CI that includes 1 is not statistically significant.

- The results are visual.

Risk

Measures of risk

New cases = incidence.
Existing cases = prevalence.

$$\text{Incidence} = \frac{\text{new illness episodes}}{\text{population at risk during a specific period of time}} \times 10^a.$$

$$\text{Prevalence} = \frac{\text{number of individuals with existing disease}}{\text{population size during specific time period}} \times 100\%.$$

Measures of association

Risk is calculated by comparing what happens to different groups of people. Consider a population that has been split into two sub-populations.

- Population 1 = population exposed to risk factor.

- Population 2 = population not exposed to risk factor.

Both populations have an associated risk of disease.

$$\text{Probability of disease/ death} = \text{Risk (R)} = \frac{\text{number with the disease}}{\text{number at risk of the disease}} = \frac{d}{n}.$$

$$\text{Risk difference (RD)} = \text{Risk1} - \text{Risk2} = \frac{d_1}{n_1} - \frac{d_2}{n_2}.$$

$$\text{Relative risk (RR)} = \frac{R_1}{R_2} = \frac{d_1/n_1}{d_2/n_2} = \frac{d_1 \times n_2}{d_2 \times n_1}.$$

$$\text{Absolute risk (AR)} = \frac{R_1 - R_2}{R_1}.$$

Absolute risk and relative risk are used to assess the strength of a relationship between a disease and any factor that might affect it.

$$\text{Absolute risk} = \frac{\text{the number of events that occur in the treated and control group}}{\text{the number of people in that group}}.$$

The absolute risk reduction is the difference between the control group and the treated group.

$$\text{ARR} = \text{ARC} - \text{ART}$$

Relative risk (or *risk ratio*) in randomised controlled trials and cohort studies, or relative odds in cohort or case-controlled studies, is the ratio of absolute risks of the disease between the two groups.

- If RR < 1, intervention reduces the risk of the outcome being studied.
- If RR = 1, the treatment has no effect on the outcome being studied.
- If RR > 1, the intervention increases the risk of the outcome being studied.

Odds

Odds are a way of representing probability. They are defined as the ratio of the probability of an event happening to that of it not happening (i.e. risk).

Odds ratio

This is a measure of the effectiveness of a treatment. It is an estimate of relative risk.

$$\text{Odds ratio} = \frac{\text{Odds in the treated group}}{\text{Odds in the control group}}.$$

- If OR < 1, the effects of the treatment are less than those of the control treatment.
- If OR = 1, the effects of the treatment are no different from those of the control treatment.
- If OR > 1, the effects of the treatment are greater than those of the control treatment.

The effects can be good or bad.

Diagnostic testing

	Disease positive	Disease negative	Total
Test positive	a	b	a + b
Test negative	c	d	c + d
Total	a + c	b + d	a + b + c + d

$$\text{Sensitivity} = \frac{\text{number of test positive and disease positive}}{\text{number of disease positive}} = \frac{a}{a + c}.$$

$$\text{Specificity} = \frac{\text{number of test negative and disease negatived}}{\text{number of disease negative}} = \frac{d}{b + d}.$$

Positive predictive value = probability that an individual who is diagnosed test positive will be a true positive

$$= \frac{a}{a+b} \cdot$$

Negative predictive value = probability that an individual who is diagnosed test negative will be a true negative

$$= \frac{d}{c+d} \cdot$$

Number needed to treat (NNT)

This is the number of people you would need to treat with a specific intervention (e.g. aspirin for people having a heart attack) to see one occurrence of a specific outcome (e.g. prevention of death).

$$NNT = \frac{1}{\text{absolute risk reduction}} \cdot$$

This value should be multiplied by 100 if using a percentage.
  Thus the smaller the absolute risk reduction the higher the NNT.

○ (2001) *J Med Screen*. **8**: 114–15.
  This paper suggests that estimates of NNT should carry a health warning. The concept of preventing one event should be compared with the more likely probability that several people will benefit by having an event delayed by a few years.
    For example, the finding that an antihypertensive drug reduces the incidence of stroke by 30% can be interpreted in two ways, namely that the drug prevented 30% of strokes (with no effect on the other 70%), or that all strokes in the treatment group were delayed by 3 years.

Other statistical terms

Bias

This is deviation of the results from the truth – a one-sided inclination of the mind.

- *publication bias* occurs when studies with positive results are more likely to be published.
- *selection bias* occurs when there are systematic differences between sample and target populations.
- *information bias* occurs when there are systematic errors in the measurement of outcome or exposure.

Heterogeneity

This term is used when there is no overlap of the trials used in a meta-analysis.

Homogeneity ('similarity')

This term is used when all trials on the plot have an overlap of confidence intervals (i.e. in a meta-analysis).

Meta-analysis

This is a paper that looks at a number of original research papers in an attempt to answer a question by summarising the findings of several papers.

Validity

This refers to how rigorous a study is.

- *Study validity* is validity with respect to internal and external bias.

- *Internal validity* is the degree to which conclusions internal to the study are legitimate.

- *External validity* is the degree to which conclusions generated from the sample could be generalised to the target population.

Study designs

Experimental study designs

- *Randomised controlled trial* – a minimum of two groups to which patient allocation is random, where one of the groups is the control (i.e. non-experimental group).

Observational study designs

- *Cross-sectional survey* – a study in which the sample frame is observed at one particular time. It gives prevalence estimates, and cause and effect are difficult to establish.

- *Cohort study* – a longitudinal follow-up of two or more cohorts (groups) with recorded exposure to a risk factor. It provides comparative incidence estimates between exposed and non-exposed groups. There can be surveillance bias.

- *Case-controlled study* – this is used to compare two groups when prevalence is low. Odds ratios are used for analysis.

Forest plot

This is a pictorial representation of Odds ratios in the form of horizontal lines. They represent the 95% confidence interval of each trial, with a vertical line representing the point where the study intervention would have no effect (i.e. if the horizontal line crosses the vertical line the result is not significant).

Funnel plot

This is a graph in which each study is represented by a dot, the position of which depends on the size of the effect of the intervention (on the horizontal axis) and the size of the study (on the vertical axis).

Part 3

Introduction

Part 3 takes a 'rounding-up' approach, including all of the remaining topics not covered in Parts 1 and 2 that are useful for general practice and the registrar year itself, as well as exam questions, whether you are taking summative assessment, the MRCGP or just refreshing your memory.

The encouragement of lifelong learning (by means of personal development plans, appraisal, revalidation, etc.) means that attitudes and approaches will be notably different as learners draw upon professional and life experiences as well as the hard facts. Adult learning is increasingly self-directed, as facts are retained better in this way than with didactic teaching. When working for the exams, I would encourage you to tackle topics individually. Read around them, discuss them and apply the knowledge you develop to everyday practice.

With regard to the exam-style questions, an explanation is given of what is involved, together with suggestions on how to tackle the questions (e.g. against the clock, in pairs, etc.). There is, of course, an overriding message – if you don't like the suggestions given here, then do them in any way that suits you. All of the answers are comprehensive but not exhaustive. As you get used to the technique and increase your knowledge base, you will find points that you consider important that are not included in the answers in this book. Depending how strongly you feel about this, feel free to email your suggestions to gear@doctors.org.uk.

GMC Duties of a Doctor

- Make the care of your patients your first concern.

- Treat every patient politely and considerately.

- Respect patient dignity and privacy.

- Listen to patients and respect their views.

- Give patients information in a form they can understand.

- Respect patients' rights to be fully involved in decisions about their care.

- Keep your professional skills and knowledge up to date.

- Recognise the limits of your professional competence.

- Be honest and trustworthy.

- Respect and protect confidential information.

- Make sure that your personal beliefs do not prejudice your patients' care.

- Act quickly to protect patients from risk if you have a good reason to believe that you or a colleague may not be fit to practise.

- Avoid abusing your position as a doctor.

- Work with colleagues in the ways that best serve your patients' interests.

In all of the above matters you must never discriminate unfairly against your patients or colleagues, and you must always be prepared to justify your actions.

○ (2002) What is a good doctor and how do you make one? *BMJ*. **324**: 556–710.
  This edition is dedicated to good performance and the qualities that contribute to being a good doctor (e.g. contentment).

WONCA European definition of general practice

WONCA is the World Organisation of Family Doctors, which published a new definition of family practice in 2002. An overview of this was published in *The New Generalist* in spring 2003.

The discipline of general practice:

- is normally the first point of medical contact in the healthcare system

- makes efficient use of resources through co-ordination

- develops a person-centred approach

- has a unique consultation process that establishes a relationship over time

- has a decision-making process that is based on the prevalence and incidence of illness

- manages acute and chronic problems

- promotes health and well-being

- deals with health problems in their physical, psychological, social, cultural and existential dimensions.

The specialty of general practice can be summarised as follows.

- GPs are specialist physicians trained in the principles of the discipline. They are primarily responsible for the provision of comprehensive and continuing care.

- They care for individuals in the context of their family, community and culture. They recognise that they have a professional responsibility to their community.

- They exercise their professional role by promoting health, preventing disease and providing cure or palliation.

They must take responsibility for maintaining their skills, personal balance and values.

Income in general practice (will become obsolete once new GP contract is in place)

The Red Book (which will be available in your practice) and *Medeconomics* (especially the back pages) are both more detailed sources of information.

NHS

- Practice allowance (dependent on list size, number of GPs and hours worked).

- Rent and rates (cost rent and notional rent).

- Rural practice allowance.

- Deprivation payment.

- Capitation fees:
  - patients (age dependent)
  - registration fee (new patient checks)
  - child health surveillance (CHS) fees (GP needs to be on CHS list, i.e. appropriately trained).

- Item-of-service fees:
  - night visits
  - contraceptive services
  - travel vaccinations.

- Maternity medical services.

- Target payments:
  - childhood immunisations (there are two levels: 70% and 90%)
  - cervical cytology (there are two levels: 50% and 80%).

- Sessional fees:
  - health promotion (diabetes, coronary heart disease, smoking, etc.)
  - minor surgery
  - medical students.

- Postgraduate education allowance.

- Seniority payments.

- Additional income:
  - clinical assistant post
  - training practice
  - dispensing practice
  - temporary residents.

- Reimbursements (water rates, staff, computers, waste, etc.).

Non-NHS

- Contract work:
  - nursing homes
  - schools
  - occupational health for local organisations.

- Insurance examinations and reports.

- Cremation fees.

- Private scripts and sick notes, etc.

Multiple-choice questions for the MRCGP and summative assessment

These papers are machine marked, and they test a huge amount of knowledge in a relatively short period of time. The papers will include medicine, management, administration issues, research, epidemiology and statistics. For this reason it is not advisable to sit the exam until you have done at least 3 months of general practice.

When you are revising, don't forget that ENT, ophthalmology, dermatology, etc., will feature in the exam.

The way to improve at multi-choice question (MCQ) exams is to answer sample questions, mark them, and then read around the questions you got wrong *and* the questions you got right because of a lucky guess.

In the MRCGP exam, do not be surprised at the number of extended matching questions on the paper. There will be instructions, and usually you have to choose the single best answer for the stem question asked. Another favourite is to have an abstract supplied with missing key words, which you then have to identify correctly from a list. Again the exam information will go through different question styles and give examples. On the day, make sure that you read the information given and the question very carefully.

For MCQ exams, it is important to know how to interpret a number of recognised phrases.

The following definitions are from the college guidelines, but you will find almost identical definitions in most MCQ books.

- *Diagnostic, characteristic, pathognomonic* or *in the vast majority* – implies that the feature would occur in 90% of cases.

- *Typically, frequently, significantly, commonly* or *in a substantial majority* – implies that the feature would occur in 60% of cases or more.

- *In the majority* – implies that the feature would occur in 50% of cases or more.

- *In the minority* – implies that the feature would occur in less than 50% of cases.

- *Low chance* or *in a substantial minority* – implies that the feature may occur in up to 30% of cases.

- *Has been shown, recognised* or *reported* – all refer to evidence found in authoritative medical texts.

Here we have included some samples of our own MCQs. We have not done a paper as such, because there is a multitude of books available.

Sample multiple-choice questions

Questions

Answer True or False for each of the following.

Dermatological emergencies include:
1 erythrasma
2 erythrodermic psoriasis
3 epidermal necrolysis
4 Norwegian scabies
5 pitted keratolysis.

Diseases that are known to koebnerise include:
6 pityriasis rosea
7 psoriasis
8 lichen sclerosis
9 lichen planus
10 erythema multiforme
11 pityriasis lichenoides.

The eyedrops below are noted for the following:
12 bradycardia is seen with pilocarpine
13 cyclopentolate can precipitate glaucoma
14 when using atropine drops for refraction, the effects can last for up to 2 months
15 exacerbation of asthma can occur with timolol
16 Rose Bengal is useful for visualising corneal ulceration.

The following are recognised as improving survival in acute myocardial infarction:
17 aspirin
18 thrombolysis given within 48 hours of onset of the pain
19 atenolol
20 nifedipine
21 immediate percutaneous transluminal angioplasty
22 warfarin.

In drug treatment of non-insulin-dependent diabetes mellitus:
23 sulphonylureas suppress appetite
24 metformin may cause hypoglycaemia
25 chlorpropramide is a suitable sulphonylurea for use in the elderly
26 thiazolidindiones are associated with liver damage
27 prandial glucose regulators are not yet licensed in the UK.

With regard to postnatal depression:
28 1 in 50 women become depressed after childbirth

29 the Edinburgh Postnatal Depression Scale is designed for use 6–8 weeks post-natally
30 postnatal depression commonly starts 3–5 days after childbirth
31 SSRIs are of proven benefit.

Diagnosis of altered bowel habit

For each patient in questions 32 to 36, select the most likely cause of the problem from the list of options below.

a   carcinoma of the colon
b   irritable bowel syndrome
c   *Campylobacter* enteritis
d   giardiasis
e   Crohn's disease
f   ischaemic colitis
g   pseudomembranous colitis
h   laxative abuse
i   chronic pancreatitis

32 An 18-year-old girl has been amenorrhoeic for 6 months, has lost a lot of weight and has developed loose stools (at least four times a day).

33 A 28-year-old woman has recently been made redundant. She has started to experience episodic diarrhoea with small-volume stools and a feeling of incomplete defecation. There is abdominal pain and bloating.

34 A 22-year-old student has returned from Russia with episodic loose stool and is passing offensive wind.

35 A 48-year-old man with a family history of polyposis coli defaulted from the surveillance programme some years ago. Over the last 3 months he has developed altered bowel habit and has lost a little weight. He has had one episode of rectal bleeding.

36 A 36-year-old businessman has completed a 2-week course of cephalexin. He has now developed a fever, diarrhoea and cramping abdominal pains.

For each of the drugs in questions 37 to 41, choose the most appropriate item from the list of options below.

a   oligogyric crisis
b   serotonin syndrome
c   exfoliative dermatitis
d   venous thrombosis
e   bradycardia
f   hypertension
g   dry mouth

37 Tamoxifen.
38 Atenolol.
39 Tolterodine (Detrusitol).
40 Fluoxetine.
41 Metoclopramide.

For each of questions 42 to 48, choose the most appropriate item from the list of options below.

a   no precautions needed
b   7
c   14
d   5
e   19
f   21
g   3

42 A patient who requires postcoital contraception has presented too late for Levonelle-2. If she has a regular 28-day cycle, up to what day is it acceptable to use an IUD?

43 Microval (a progestogen-only contraceptive) is started on day 1 of your patient's period. For how many days should she use additional contraception?

44 A patient is 4 hours late taking her Loestrin 20 contraceptive pill. For how many days are extra precautions required?

45 Your patient is changing from a combined contraceptive pill to Noriday, without a break between pill packs. For how many days are extra precautions required?

46 Your patient is breastfeeding and requires contraception. How many days postpartum can the progestogen-only pill Femulen be started?

47 If your postpartum patient in the previous question wanted to start Micronor (her usual progestogen-only pill), when could this be started from?

48 Within how many days after unprotected sexual intercourse should Levonelle-2 be taken if it is to be effective as postcoital contraception?

The Mental Health Act

For each of the statements in questions 49 to 55, choose the most appropriate section from the list of options below.

a   Section 2
b   Section 3
c   Section 4

d   Section 5
e   Section 7
f   Section 12
g   Section 135
h   Section 136

49 This is used for the assessment of a patient for up to 28 days.

50 This is used only in an emergency.

51 This can be used by the police to detain a person whom they believe is suffering from a mental illness.

52 This is used for compulsory treatment of a patient with an established diagnosis.

53 This is appropriate for guardianship.

54 This gives the police right of entry into private premises to remove a patient to a place of safety.

55 this is used to approve doctors who are recognised as having specialised expertise in mental health.

Medical statistics

Match each of the statements in questions 56 to 60 with the most appropriate term from the list of options below.
a   correlation
b   confidence
c   incidence
d   predictive value
e   confounding

56 This depends on the sensitivity and specificity of a test.

57 This needs to be eliminated in a reliable study.

58 This depends on the prevalence of a disease in the population studied.

59 This is the occurrence of new cases in a population over a given period of time.

60 This occurs when a variable changes in a way that is directly related to another variable.

Hypertension screening

	Screening test positive	Screening test negative
Hypertension present	340	51
Hypertension not present	82	172

For each of the items in questions 61 to 65, select the most appropriate answer from the list of options below.

a   51/391
b   51/223
c   340/391
d   340/422
e   82/254
f   82/422
g   172/223
h   172/254
i   340
j   51
k   82
l   172

61 Specificity.

62 Sensitivity.

63 Positive predictive value.

64 Negative predictive value.

65 False negative.

Hip screening test performed in neonates

	Screening test positive	Screening test negative
Problem present	29	42
Problem absent	64	364

For each of the items in questions 66 to 70, choose the most appropriate answer from the list of options below.

a 29/93
b 29/71

c 42/71
d 42/408
e 64/93
f 64/428
g 364/408
h 364/428
i 29
j 51
k 64
l 364

66 Positive predictive value.

67 Negative predictive value.

68 Specificity.

69 Sensitivity.

70 False negative.

Answers

 1 False
 2 True
 3 True
 4 False
 5 False

 6 False
 7 True
 8 True
 9 True
10 True
11 False

12 False (seen with beta-blocker drops)
13 True (it is mydriatic)
14 False (2 weeks)
15 True
16 True

17 True
18 False (needs to be within 24 hours)
19 True (ISIS 1)
20 False

21 False (significant mortality)
22 False

23 False (they stimulate insulin secretion, so stimulate appetite)
24 False (sulphonylureas do)
25 False (this has the longest half-life; tolbutamide would be a better option)
26 True (troglitazone was withdrawn because of this)
27 False

28 False (1 in 10)
29 True
30 False (commonly 4–6 weeks; baby blues 3–5 days)
31 True (as are tricyclic antidepressants)

32 h
33 b
34 d
35 a
36 g

37 d
38 e
39 g
40 b
41 a

42 e
43 c
44 a
45 a
46 b
47 f
48 g

49 a
50 c
51 h
52 b
53 e
54 g
55 f

56 d
57 e
58 d
59 c
60 a

61 h
62 c
63 d
64 g
65 j

66 a
67 g
68 h
69 b
70 j

The written paper

The main aim of the written paper is to examine your ability to integrate and apply theoretical knowledge and professional values within the setting of primary healthcare in the UK.

The written paper is an arm-cramping three and a half hours long, but not one person coming out of the exam has been heard to claim that they had plenty of time. Make sure you have done at least one past paper against the clock. Past papers can be downloaded from the college website, including the critical reading sections (www.rcgp.org.uk). Unfortunately, there are no model answers, just examiners' comments, but past papers are still a must.

Excluding the critical reading questions, this paper is mainly about your ability to problem solve. As in real life, the most important aspect is not knowing all the answers, but asking the right questions along the way, and taking the time to explore all of the options.

The two most important things you need to look at are:

1 the exam regulations and notes
2 past papers from the college website (www.rcgp.org.uk).

The following suggestions might help you in preparing for the exam.

- Keep up to date. This goes for all areas of the exam, as well as at work.

- Consider taking part in a study group. You can cover much more ground, and it helps to keep you motivated. Look at hot topics, GP issues, questions, etc.

- Practise against the clock, and try to keep to 15 minutes for each question.

- Try to structure your answers rather than writing freestyle. It helps you to think and the examiner to mark more quickly (so is less frustrating for them).

- Think broadly, and try to include ethical and cultural issues as well as personal development points.

- A course is not a necessity. Before you choose and pay for one, try to find people who have been on a course, as some are better than others.

Below we have set out a 'paper', consisting of 12 questions, that does not include any critical reading.

In this section we suggest that you give yourself a maximum of 3 hours for the 12 questions. If at all possible, try to treat it as a mock exam, as this will get you used to formulating and writing your answers quickly. We have included a section on the process of critical reading, and we really do advocate that on a regular basis you practise this to improve both your skills and your speed. There are also several very simply written books on critical reading, and if your library does not stock these already, they may be willing to purchase them. If not, they are easy to get hold of.

The answers are printed below the questions. It is all too easy to take a sneaky look at the answers, and then you will be left not knowing what you really do know and where your gaps are. Compare your answers with our own and those of your colleagues, friends and even your trainer.

If you make it to the end (or get bored), then make up some of your own problem-based questions. Try keeping a list of problems or heartsinks from work. This may help you to understand the issues, and your heartsink may become a success story. This is one method to take forward for your personal development plan. The exam is not about catching you out, but about testing your approach to real problems that you may encounter in everyday practice.

Written question 1

You are asked to take a call by your receptionist. A young mother is wanting advice about her 8-year-old son who has a cold and has developed a blotchy red rash. How do you deal with such a request?

This question is testing your approach to telephone consultations. This is an expanding role in general practice, and if handled incorrectly the consequences can be disastrous.

The telephone consultation lends itself to Neighbour's consultation model.

1 Introduce yourself.

2 Establish who you are speaking to and who is the patient.

3 Establish a rapport, do not rush, actively listen, and ask questions to clarify.

4 Summarise.

5 Agree a plan.

6 Safety net (this is very important).

7 Make accurate records at the time, and do not forget to date and time the entry.

Practice points

- Triaging of calls: receptionist, nurse, duty doctor.
  - What would be the safest method and make the best use of time?

- Role of the nurses.
  - Is there a need for expansion of their role with regard to triage?
  - Is there an individual wish for their roles to expand?

- Accessibility of the doctor.
  - For emergencies only or immediate access?
  - For enquiries (call back/telephone access) is it worth setting aside a particular time of the day when patients know that they can phone?
  - Would increased accessibility improve patient satisfaction ?

- Is there a need for protocols:
  - for access
  - for triage
  - for telephone consultations.

Doctor issues

- Duty to patients.
  - Accessible and convenient.
  - If you are not happy, do not compromise patient safety, but arrange to see the patient.
  - Medical point: is there a need to make a diagnosis, determine what over-the-counter remedies, etc. have been tried?

- Workload.
  - Telephone accessibility may reduce the number of appointments/home visits needed.
  - It may be time-consuming to get the notes, check the information, and ensure that the patient really does understand any issues which you feel are important.

- Telephone consultation skills.
  - These need to be good (clear understanding, management plan, safety netting, etc.).
  - Be fully aware of the risks of misunderstanding.
  - Increased patient and doctor satisfaction if done well.

- Learning needs.
  - Develop consultation skills.
  - Audit of outcomes.
  - Record-keeping, etc.

- Stress.
  - This may increase (paranoia of being wrong) as well as decrease (one less patient to see).

- Prescribing issues.
    - A multitude of issues are raised when you have not seen the patient.

- Education.
    - Ongoing personal development of such skills.

Patient issues

- Why are they phoning?
    - Are there appointment problems, etc.?
- If they are just phoning for advice, are they aware of NHS Direct?

Other issues

- NHS Direct role.
    - Advertise in surgery (advice line for minor illnesses).
- Pharmacists.
    - Roles are expanding, especially in over-the-counter self-management.
- Public Health.
    - Advertising campaigns for self-management of minor self-limiting illnesses.
- Cultural and social factors (e.g. access to a telephone, language barriers, etc.).

Written question 2

How would you explain a diagnosis of IBS (irritable bowel syndrome) to a patient? You have made the diagnosis on the basis of history (ROME II criteria), normal examination and investigation.

Irritable bowel syndrome is the most common functional gastrointestinal problem seen in practice.

There is no known cause, and it is likely to have a multi-factoral aetiology.

Common factors that can affect IBS include the following:

- diet, although not because of allergy

- stress (in more than 50% of patients)

- gastrointestinal infections (e.g. following *Campylobacter* infection).

The diagnosis would need to be discussed sensitively, rather than dismissively, given the probable degree of symptoms.

Give the patient chance to ask questions. In particular, explore his or her own ideas and concerns.

How might IBS affect a patient's life?

These areas need to be considered individually.

- Pain.
  - This is mainly due to abdominal bloating, although haemorrhoids can develop secondary to straining.
  - IBS patients tend to have a lower pain threshold (clinically proven in trials).

- Psychological factors.
  - Anxiety or depression may be a trigger or a resultant factor.
  - Chronic pain is known to affect psychological morbidity.

- Work-related factors.
  - Pain may impair performance or make work impossible (i.e. the disorder has socio-economic implications).

- Family life.
  - If pain and unpredictability of the symptoms are long-standing, this may affect relationships (e.g. psychological aspects, dyspareunia, etc.).

What treatment has been proven to be of benefit?

- Antispasmodics:
  - mebeverine (NNT = 6) (inhibits intestinal smooth muscle contraction)
  - hyoscine (NNT = 9) (anticholinergic effects).

- Bulking agents:
  - ispaghula husk (NNT = 4).

- Anti-diarrhoeal agents:
  - loperamide (NNT = 3).

- Antidepressants (not for antidepressant effect):
  - low-dose tricyclics (NNT = 3)
  - $5HT_4$ agonists (improve constipation)
  - $5HT_3$ antagonists (reduce diarrhoea).

These figures have been taken from the Primary Care Society for Gastroenterology guidelines.

- Complementary therapy:
  - hypnosis, cognitive behavioural therapy, biofeedback and psychotherapy have all been reported to be useful in certain cases
  - relaxation techniques, Chinese herbal medicine and acupuncture may also help, but as yet no convincing data have been published to support the claims.

When explaining the diagnosis, it is important to discuss the management options and develop a plan together with the patient.

Written question 3

You are given the role of improving diabetic care in your practice. How would you tackle the project?

It is known that lack of structure increases mortality in diabetic care, so organisation of services is of great importance.

With the recent publication of the Delivery Strategy for the National Service Framework for diabetes and the implications of the New Contract, this is an important area to have in order.

Determine the objectives

- Patient groups to be targeted:
  - NIDDM
  - IDDM
  - diet-controlled diabetes and impaired glucose tolerance
  - screening issues
  - coronary heart disease groups.

- Look at the evidence base and Government guidelines on what goals should be, especially with regard to the following:
  - blood pressure control (HOT study)
  - HbA_{1C} targets (UKPDS 33)
  - chiropody and ophthalmology checks
  - weight, obesity, diet and exercise
  - cholesterol and lipids.

Need to co-ordinate with secondary care where possible

Practice meeting to include all people to be involved clinically

- Develop objectives.

- Write guidelines or adopt previously written ones.

- Write leaflets or adopt previously written ones.

- Protocols depending on nurse involvement – they may wish to take the lead.

- Appointment system and clinic set-up (computer recall and template use for recall).

Audit current standards

- This should include a patient questionnaire on quality and satisfaction.

- Implement changes and set time scales.

- Re-audit (i.e. complete the audit cycle).

Significant event analysis

- Problems from clinic.

- Management points to be learned from mistakes.

Depending on your practice population, be aware of cultural issues and have appropriate advice to hand (e.g. on Ramadan).

Further issues

- Funding, equipment, register.

- Take into account the holistic approach:
  - flu and pneumococcal counselling
  - psychological impact of the disease
  - pre-conceptual counselling, etc.

What evidence is there to support aggressive blood pressure control in diabetes?

- Around 70% of patients with NIDDM have hypertension.

- There is a known increase in the risk of cardiovascular disease, myocardial infarction, cerebrovasular accident, nephropathy and retinopathy in diabetics. This risk is significantly increased if there is concurrent hypertension.

- British Hypertension Society guidelines recommend that treated blood pressure in diabetics should be <140/80 mmHg. The threshold for starting treatment is ⩾140/90.

- Blood pressure reduction in diabetes has been shown to reduce the incidence of cardiovascular events and mortality.

○ (1998) SHEP diabetic subgroup. *Arch Intern Med.* **158**: 741–51.

○ (1998) HOT study
Blood pressure of 130/80 mmHg reduced events by up to 50%. *Lancet.* **351**: 1755–62.

○ Micro-HOPE study.
Treatment with an ACE inhibitor (ramipril), although the study was not specifically looking at a hypertensive population, showed a reduction in cardiovascular events and overt nephropathy. Although a reduction in blood pressure was part of the effect, it is thought that there is also a reno-protective effect of ramipril/ACE inhibitors.

○ UKPDS.
Lowering systolic blood pressure reduces the incidence of myocardial infarction and cerebrovascular accident by up to 44%. The lowest risk is seen with a systolic blood pressure of <120 mmHg. There are suggestions that lowering blood pressure is of more benefit than glucose control.

○ SYST-EUR (SHEP Co-operative Research Group from 1988 and 1997).
The excess risk of diabetes was virtually eliminated with antihypertensive treatment.

Written question 4

You receive a health authority circular about a patient who is suspected of attempting to obtain drugs such as dihydrocodeine and temazepam under various different names, usually as a temporary resident.

As you read through the circular, it becomes increasingly apparent that you have probably seen the woman and issued her with the drugs.

How would you deal with the situation?

Seeing temporary residents and issuing drugs for patients with whom you are not familiar is a relatively common scenario. In this case it would appear that someone is defrauding the system and putting herself, and maybe others, at risk.

Patient issues

- Why do the drugs need to be obtained deceitfully (i.e. what gains are in this for the patient)?
  - because of over-use and dependence?
  - for their retail value?
  - for another person who is dependent?

- Can she be contacted (has she given a fake address and telephone number) in order to exclude her from the inquiry, or to confirm her involvement?

- Is there any drug dependence or criminal history (i.e. is this a repeat offence or a new problem that is amenable to help)?

- Psychological state – the patient will need full assessment; are there other under-lying medical or psychiatric problems?

Doctor issues

You need to be as certain as possible that this could be the same patient.

- Confidentiality.
  - You have a duty of care to this patient, even if she is a temporary resident, who needs help.
  - The GMC guidelines on confidentiality state that you can disclose information if the patient poses a serious risk to him- or herself or others.
  - Disclose only what is necessary (e.g. you may not need to mention the medical reasons for requesting the treatment).

- Defence organisation – it is important, if you have any doubts, to discuss with your defence union what it would be prudent to disclose.

- Who to inform:
  - the health authority contact
  - the police who are dealing with the case

- other partners and reception staff
- other practices in the area if they have not received the circular.

- Written account – it is important to keep your own written account for future reference.
  - If this case ends up in court, you may be asked for more information than you put on your statement.

- Personal development issues:
  - you need to be aware of, and discuss if necessary, feelings of betrayal, etc.
  - were you singled out for any particular reason?
  - do you have a mentor?

Practice issues

- Temporary residents.
  - All forms should be fully completed.
  - If NHS numbers, etc., are not known, should the patient's own GP be contacted for the information prior to the patient being seen?
  - Should doctors repeat prescribe for temporary residents? This is not a simple 'yes or no' issue. Should certain drugs be excluded?
  - Practice development issues.

- Computer.
  - All patients should be input, so creating a trail.

- Prescriptions.
  - Avoid handwritten scripts altogether if possible.
  - If prescribing is done by computer, this creates a trail.

- Significant event analysis.
  - Is this a case you could all learn from?

- Consider audit.
  - On temporary residents.
  - Any repeat visits?

- Use of the Internet to confirm GPs and address supplied.
  - www.gpinfo.com
  - www.streetmap.co.uk

Written question 5

In the light of the new strategy for sexual health, what implications would HIV testing have in primary care?

Approximately 30 000 people in the UK have HIV, and this number is still rising. The sexual health strategy recommends that all GPs should offer HIV counselling and testing. Currently less than 1% of practices offer this service (7% in London).

Routine screening in pregnancy is already offered in virtually all areas. This tends to be blanket screening, rather than identifying the population at increased risk. It has the obvious benefit that if the patient is HIV-positive, and this is discovered before birth and early on in the pregnancy, it is possible to prevent or reduce transmission to the foetus from 20–30% to 2%.

Doctor and practice issues

- Improved and extended service for patients.

- Improved communication (i.e. GPs are more likely to be aware if their patients are on treatment for HIV, and can alter their other prescribing accordingly).

- Education and training (counselling skills, current treatment for HIV and AIDS, etc.):
  - what sort of advice to be giving (shaving, tooth brushing, what to do if the patient cuts him- or herself, etc.)
  - need to be aware of associated drug misuse and the implications of this for management and transmission of the disease.

- Workload implications:
  - time for screening and counselling
  - arranging for samples to be taken in an anonymous fashion if required
  - dealing with positive results (i.e. referral if necessary)
  - ensuring that repeat tests are performed where necessary
  - other swabs that need doing or hepatitis B status (especially if it is late on Friday night and the patient is unlikely to return, which will mean swabs sitting around all weekend)
  - contact tracing, and who will take the responsibility if the patient will not?

- Confidentiality issues.
  - If samples are not labelled anonymously, anyone can see the names.
  - If you obtain a positive result and the patient will not inform their partner(s), especially if their partner is a patient of yours.

- Improved job satisfaction as skills and service develop.

- Resources:
  - GP, nurse and phlebotomy time
  - cost of the tests, administration and follow-up
  - if diagnosed early, morbidity and mortality can be dramatically decreased with treatment. This will mean higher drug costs for a longer period of time.

- Audit (i.e. appointment uptake/DNA rate):
  - positive results (is screening being performed appropriately?)
  - outcome and patient satisfaction.

Primary healthcare team issues

- What would be their level of involvement?
- Counselling by community psychiatric nurse if there is a positive result.
- Dentist – again if positive, as only certain dentists will accept HIV-positive patients.
- Nurses – general all-round input, especially at the AIDS stage of the disease.

Patient issues

- Increased accessibility for patients – general practice is generally much more accessible than secondary care.
- Increased patient satisfaction.
- Improved doctor–patient relationship because of GP involvement.
- Patient may lack confidence in:
  - GP knowledge, because GPs are generalists, not specialists
  - confidentiality within the practice.
- Improved long-term outcome (i.e. reduction in mortality and morbidity).
- Improved quality of life.

Cultural and language barriers

- You need to consider patients' needs:
  - whether an interpreter needs to be employed – this has associated confidentiality issues
  - gender problems – a female patient may not consent to be seen by a male doctor, and vice versa, for swabs, etc.

Secondary care implications

- Would free up appointments for more complicated patients, so that GPs would be able to access secondary care more easily when a result is positive.
- Improved shared care and interprofessional relationships.
- There may be a need for guidelines for HIV management, drawn up by both primary and secondary care physicians.

Written question 6

Margaret is a 66-year-old woman who retired 18 months ago from running an excellent nursing home in the area. She was diagnosed shortly afterwards with ovarian cancer (for which she had nursed her sister).

On seeing her today, despite morphine treatment, her abdominal pain is becoming increasingly difficult to control. What can you do to help her?

The World Health Organization definition of palliative care is as follows:

The active total care of patients whose disease is not responsive to curative treatment. Control of pain, of other symptoms and of psychological, social and spiritual problems is paramount. The goal of palliative care is achievement of the best quality of life for patients and their families.

There is a lot to offer this woman in terms of active treatment. One of the most valuable things you can give her is your time. Listen to her explanation of symptoms and worries and her story.

Patient issues

- You need to allow this patient time to express her 'ideas, concerns and expectations'.

- The psychological impact of having nursed her sister with the same disease, and no doubt patients with terminal problems at the nursing home where she worked, will have probably left her with a lot of preconceived ideas and worries.
  - Is there any depression or anxiety because of the disease, the pain or other issues?
  - Does she think that pain equals progression of the cancer?

- What support is there?
  - Is she trying to protect those close to her and bottling up everything that is worrying her, so that she is left feeling isolated?

- Has she thought about death (more than likely)?
  - The pain may mean that this has been on her mind more than ever, and she is possibly fearing the event.
  - What sort of death did her sister have?
  - It may be that fear is increasing her perception of the pain.

- Social and financial issues.
  - Does she have financial worries or support?
  - If she still has a mortgage, can this be paid off?
  - Are friends reluctant to visit or visiting too much?

- Spiritual feelings.
  - Often beliefs become more significant as death approaches.
  - Does she need any help with contacting the appropriate minister?

- Legal issues.
  - Is she prepared?
  - Has she made a will? (Is she aware of issues like inheritance tax?).

Doctor issues

- Pain – on the face of it this is the main issue, and it needs to be fully explored as appropriate.
  - 80% of cancer patients have more than one type of pain
  - 30% have more than three types.

- History and examination:
  - ?ascites (needs tapping)
  - ?jaundice (liver capsule pain)
  - ?tumour bulk
  - ?bony metastases
  - ?subacute bowel obstruction

Presumably the patient's suitability for chemotherapy, radiotherapy and surgery was assessed and discussed at the time of diagnosis. Sometimes it is worth reconsidering the options.

- Conventional treatment:
  - increased analgesia (oral, patch, subcutaneous, etc.)
  - anti-emetics or laxatives may be necessary
  - antidepressants, steroids, dietary supplements etc.

- Complementary treatment:
  - acupuncture
  - relaxation therapy
  - homeopathy etc.

- Legal issues.
  - Have the issues of resuscitation or advance directive been discussed?

- Confidentiality.
  - Although there may be family around, the patient may not want to involve them – be aware of this.

- Accessibility.
  - Who will provide palliative care out of hours? Will it be you or your local co-operative?
  - Communication is essential if care is to be handed over.
  - Is there a practice policy on palliative care? Does there need to be one?
  - Accessibility to other services in the primary healthcare team is also important.

- Bereavement counselling:
  - for both Margaret and her family.

- Cultural and ethical issues surrounding her care.
  - What treatment does she and doesn't she want (autonomy, non-maleficence)?
  - How does she want to die? Are there any special requests for how her body is treated, etc.?

- Personal implications.
  - You have to deal with your own grief.
  - Such cases can take up a lot of time, which can be either fulfilling/rewarding or irritating.
  - Housekeeping is very important (e.g. talking to partners).

Primary healthcare team issues

- Macmillan nurse involvement (if it has not already been sought, now might be a good time).
- District nurse (e.g. for support, syringe drivers, enemas, etc.).
- Physiotherapy (for maintaining mobility, loan of TENS machine, acupuncture, etc.).
- Community psychiatric nurse (if considered helpful in the situation is a useful resource).
- Social services:
  - DS1500 and benefits
  - home aids (also occupational therapy).

Written question 7

A woman attends for a pill check. As you are taking her blood pressure you notice various bruises up her arm.
   How would you tackle such a finding?

This is a question on domestic violence. Although in this case you are witness to what seems to be the physical manifestation of abuse, always be aware of the emotional and mental aspects, too.

Up to 25% of women will experience domestic violence at some point in their life. Although this question deals with a woman, men can suffer similar abuse, although there are no accurate statistics (the numbers are thought to be lower). It is a problem that is under-identified in the UK for a multitude of reasons.

Patient issues

- Is this her (not so) hidden agenda? (She would have known about the bruises and that you would have to take her blood pressure.)
- Does she have low self-esteem, depression, anxiety, etc.?
- Are you her last resort? What has she tried up until now?
- Are there children involved? Are they at risk? Do social services, health visitors or the child protection team need to be informed and involved?

- What other fears does she have?
  - social isolation
  - financial worries
  - her own anger and ability to exact revenge
  - the risk of permanent injury
  - the safety and well-being of her children
  - the shame of people finding out, etc.

Doctor issues

- A good place to start is to ask.

○ (2002) Bradley *et al*. *BMJ*. **324**: 271–4.
  This study found that most women welcome enquiries but that doctors and nurses rarely ask. It also found that there was a strong association with anxiety and depression.

- Make a thorough assessment of the patient:
  - physical and psychological factors, alcohol and drug use
  - social history, support and current situation.

- Confidentiality – this is an important point to emphasise.

- Notes.
  - You need excellent documentation of any injuries witnessed, a history of events (if this is forth-coming) and your assessment.
  - Consider medical illustration for photographic evidence.

- Learning needs.
  - Is this an area you need to brush up on?
  - It raises issues such as communication skills, ethics and human rights.
  - Are you aware of the local services available so that you are able to advise the patient about them?

- Accessibility.
  - This woman needs a point of contact (e.g. the police, Women's Aid National Helpline, etc.) if she runs into further problems.

- Is the abusing partner a patient of yours?
  - Are there psychological, anger or alcohol-related problems that you could help with in order to improve the situation?

Practice issues

- Is there a need for a practice protocol and update on domestic violence?

- Is written information available?
  - This is mainly about helplines (be aware of the implications if this material is found at home).
  - Should this information be displayed on a noticeboard/in the toilets (male as well as female)?

- Screening is an issue that is repeatedly raised. We know that patients who are affected want to be asked, and that those who are not affected do not mind being asked. Tact and diplomacy are helpful attributes. The issue of screening raises numerous points. For example:
  - time (another thing to screen for in a 10-minute consultation)
  - selective screening (on clinical suspicion)
  - training (in communication skills)
  - the abuse may involve rape and meticulous collection of samples (involvement of a police surgeon would be needed).

- ○ (2002) Could health professionals screen women for domestic violence? Systematic review. *BMJ.* **324**: 314–18.
  This review found that 50–75% of women felt that screening was acceptable. Only 30% of family doctors (mostly in American studies) felt that it was acceptable. Only two studies showed a decrease in physical and non-physical abuse as a result of intervention. It was concluded that it would be premature to introduce screening at this stage.

Primary healthcare team issues

- Role of community psychiatric nurse.
- The health visitor and social services may be aware, or may need to be informed (especially with regard to child welfare).

Written question 8

A young Chinese student has recently registered with your practice, having come to the UK with her husband in order to study. She comes to you requesting some more of her herbal medicine which she was given for pelvic pain and 'narrowed tubes'. How would you deal with this situation?

The boundaries between alternative and Western conventional medicine are becoming less clearly defined. It is just as important to understand herbal medicines and their side-effects as it is for any other drug. Unfortunately, reliable literature on some treatments is hard to come by.

Patient issues

You need to explore this woman's history further.

- What was previously investigated and what did she understand (e.g. sexually transmitted diseases, pelvic inflammatory disease, infertility, etc.)?
- What exactly is she taking and for what purpose?
- Are she and her husband trying to conceive? If so, is the remedy teratogenic? Should she stop using it altogether? It is important to counsel her appropriately.
- How is she funding her study?

- Are there financial problems? Is this why she has turned to you for a script?

- Is there a second reason for coming to the UK? Is there a hidden medical agenda?

Doctor issues

- Is it possible to access medical records (with the patient's consent)?

- Is it necessary to repeat certain tests (e.g. swabs, ultrasound scans, laparoscopy and dye, etc.)?

- If you are not familiar with the treatment and there are no medical issues that you need to address, is there a reputable Chinese herbalist in the area whom you can recommend to her? This would depend on the patient's wish for treatment as well as her ability to afford it.

Cultural ideals

Be aware of the cultural differences, particularly in terms of health, diagnosis and treatments. Not all countries are as strict as the UK about requiring documentation before you can set up in practice, and this has a knock-on effect on what patients come to expect.

Ethical principles

Treating patients who are taking other medications can lead to problems. Although the patient's autonomy is to be respected, if you are not familiar with the treatment, how can you be sure that you are not doing your patient harm?

Written question 9

You receive a discharge letter about the death of Fred, an elderly patient, from a haemorrhagic stroke. Fred had been on warfarin for atrial fibrillation, which you had diagnosed and started treatment for 3 years previously.
  What implications does this death have?

Atrial fibrillation increases the risk of stroke. Several trials have shown that anticoagulation in this group can decrease the risk of stroke by up to 70%, but there are risks and management implications of anticoagulation therapy. Not only that, there has been at least one meta-analysis which advocates the use of aspirin over warfarin (in non-rheumatic atrial fibrillation) in terms of outcome and iatrogenic complications.

The patient's family

- Find out whether they would like (from yourself or another doctor at the practice):

- a bereavement visit
- an explanation of the treatment Fred was on (discussed openly, not in a defensive manner), and also why treatment was started.

- Listen to their worries/concerns:
  - about the stroke, treatment, and circumstances of death
  - about their grief
  - about any potential issues; try to pre-empt any complaint.

Doctor issues

- Review the individual case.
  - Was treatment appropriate and considered in full by the doctor and patient? Was this documented?
  - Was the warfarin well monitored and controlled?
  - Had there been any prescribing issues that might have potentiated the effects of the warfarin?
  - Was Fred of sound mind (i.e. taking his tablets appropriately and not likely to overdose)?
  - Were there any other untreated risk factors (e.g. hypertension, mitral stenosis, etc.)?

- If there are any discrepancies, are they worthy of a significant event analysis?

- You need to acknowledge your own sense of guilt and responsibility, especially if you had gone out of your way to convince the patient that warfarin was a good thing.

- Personal ethics of such a situation (i.e. non-maleficence).
  - Ethics are always interesting to explore. Although this patient was treated and advised for the correct reasons, the outcome is not what one would want.

Practice issues

- Is there a policy (and if not, does there need to be one?) for the following:
  - when to consider warfarin?
  - monitoring warfarin (a register of who doses the patient)
  - auditing compliance
  - auditing outcome (e.g. mortality).

- Complaints procedure.
  - Although treatment was (presumably) justified, it would be an appropriate time to update the complaints procedure and educate staff appropriately.

Primary healthcare team issues

- Consider their roles in the following:
  - bereavement within the family (e.g. community psychiatric nurse, district nurse, health visitor)

- monitoring bloods (district nurse/phlebotomist)
- elderly health checks (i.e. dementia issues); as a doctor doing a drug review/ consultation, we are easily fooled into believing that a patient has their wits about them, when it could be a completely different story at home.

Written question 10

One of your receptionists comes through red-faced to tell you that a patient of the practice is being verbally aggressive and threatening physical violence if she is not seen by a doctor immediately. There are no notes on the patient, as she has only joined the practice recently, having moved into the area.

What issues does this raise?

This is quite obviously a question about safety, violence and aggression. Violence in general practice has been on the increase. There are various theories as to why this is so, including modern-day life stresses, increased patient expectations, alcohol and drugs.

A Medical Defence Union survey found that two-thirds of doctors feared that they might be physically assaulted at work. Out of 1044 respondents, 23% had been physically assaulted over the last 5 years.

This has prompted a Government 'NHS zero tolerance campaign', which was launched in October 1999. It set a target to reduce the incidence of violence by 20% by 2001 and by 30% by 2003.

Primary care trusts should offer a safe place for doctors to see violent patients. In some areas, co-operatives are employing doctors to provide this service.

Patient issues

- Why does this patient need to see a doctor so urgently?

- Why has she moved to the area?

- Are there psychological or dependence issues (e.g. alcohol or drugs)?

- Does she have children? If so, is her violence an indication that they could be at risk?

- Is this a typical pattern of behaviour for this patient?

- Is this patient aware of your policy on violence and aggression? (It is possible that this is a way of expressing frustration, and that she in fact has learning difficulties, i.e. cannot read – not that this should be used to excuse the behaviour.)

Practice issues

As employers we are responsible for ensuring that our staff are safe at work. The Health and Safety Act 1974 highlights the need for risk assessment and training.

- Layout of the room (involvement of the police with security issues):
  - door opening outwards
  - positioning and type of furniture
  - sharps, needles, equipment, etc. kept out of sight
  - panic buttons easily accessible.

- Protocols:
  - on safety issues (zero tolerance?)
  - training (signs to look for, methods to use to dissipate tension)
  - involvement of other members of staff (e.g. chaperone)
  - involve the primary healthcare team and primary care trust, and possibly the police.

- Security:
  - consider CCTV
  - personal alarms
  - panic buttons
  - avoid unnecessary danger (e.g. having only one member of staff on duty).

- Significant event analysis.
  - Is it worthwhile using this particular case?
  - Involve all, using the session for education and debriefing.

- Training:
  - communication (could such a situation have been avoided? – non-aggressive conflict resolution)
  - break-away techniques
  - signs of pending violence.

- Review the appointment system.
  - Is this at fault? Are too few appointments causing frustration for staff as well as for patients?

- Environment.
  - Try to have a comfortable waiting-area with points of interest (other than a call-screen)

- Information.
  - Keep patients informed of delays.
  - Share among staff information about dangerous patients. If patients are violent or aggressive, they forgo some of the rights to confidentiality for the sake of the safety of your staff.

Doctor issues

- Safety for yourself, your staff and other patients is paramount. Do the police need to be called in this situation?

- Most people will settle down if they get to see a doctor, but:
  - is it safe to see this person alone?
  - do you need a chaperone?

- Be aware of safety issues.
  - Remove potential missiles or hazards (e.g. tie, stethoscope, sharps, etc.).
  - Install panic buttons.
  - Again, consider room layout. Try to make sure that the patient is not between you and the door.

- You need make a medical and psychiatric assessment.
  - What is the problem (unlikely to be a true emergency)?
  - Is it a workable problem?

- You need excellent negotiating and communication skills:
  - especially if the patient is requesting something you are not prepared to do
  - is this a learning need?

- You need to document well (consider note tagging).

- Do you feel it necessary to remove the patient, in the name of zero tolerance? If so, this would have implications for:
  - other practices in the area
  - her attitude towards doctors in the future, etc.
  If you do decide to remove the patient from your list you need to contact the police before the primary care trust in order to obtain an incident number. If you don't, the 7-day rule will apply and the patient will be entitled to medical services within that time.

- You have a duty of care to this patient both medically and ethically, but not at the expense of safety.

Miscellaneous issues

- You need to consider the implications of the effects of such behaviour on other patients, possibly reinforcing the notion that aggression works.

- Be aware of the Criminal Injuries Compensation Authority and the NHS Benefit Scheme.

Written question 11

A male patient has been discharged after having had a heart attack. There is no discharge letter, but you know from your pre-admission ECG that he had an anterior myocardial infarction.

What advice would you give him and what treatment would you want him to be on?

With recent advances in secondary prevention, there has been a significant reduction in both morbidity and mortality after myocardial infarction.

Advice

Lifestyle issues

- Smoking – if the patient is a smoker, this could be just the event to encourage him to stop. Enquire, advise and use the practice or a local QUIT clinic (or the equivalent) in conjunction with nicotine replacement therapy, etc.

- Exercise – following myocardial infarction the patient will probably be in a cardiac rehabilitation programme. Meta-analyses have shown that they can reduce mortality by 20–24%. If they are not in such a programme, the patient needs a graded exercise approach which should be maintained, to reduce blood pressure and coronary heart disease. www.cardiacrehabilitation.org.uk

- Driving – usually the patient is prohibited from driving for 6 weeks. They need to take advice (from their insurance company, the DVLA, etc.) on their fitness to drive at the end of that period (consider the possibility of heart failure, angina, etc.).
    If they hold an HGV licence, they will need an exercise tolerance test prior to being recertified.

- Diet – this advice will depend on BMI, cholesterol levels, glucose levels etc. Omega-3 oils and a Mediterranean diet are known to be beneficial and to reduce cholesterol levels. If the BMI is high, there needs to be some calorie control.

- Alcohol – should only be consumed in moderation. In excess it can increase blood pressure and cholesterol levels.

- Work – this will depend on the patient's job (i.e. whether it is manual or seden- tary). Usually they will need at least 6 weeks off work. Be aware of self- employed patients, as they will be keen to start work as soon as possible and may inadvertently put themselves at risk.

Also consider discussing and advising on psychological impact, psychosexual effect, etc.

Treatment

Postmyocardial infarction patients are six times more likely to die than age-matched controls. Further preventative treatment is therefore important.

- Aspirin

  ○ Antiplatelet Trialists' Collaboration (1994) Overview of randomised trials of antiplatelet therapy. *BMJ.* **308**: 81–106.
  This showed a 25% reduction in vascular events with aspirin (75–325 mg) in secondary prevention. The ISIS 2 trial had similar reductions.

- Beta-blockers – if there are no contraindications (e.g. asthma, hypotension, bradycardia). The ISIS 1 trial showed a benefit, with decrease in mortality, repeat infarction and sudden death (partly due to anti-arrhythmic properties).

- Statins

  ○ (1994) 4S Study. *Lancet*. **344**: 1383–9.
  This study showed that reducing cholesterol levels by 30% reduced mortality. There are several other trials that support this finding. The benefit of reducing cholesterol levels is seen even if the cholesterol is 'normal'. Diet should be tackled, usually in the first instance.

- ACE inhibitors – ISIS 4 showed a reduction in mortality.
  Patients with heart failure or with a low ejection fraction will benefit the most. The SAVE (Survival and Ventricular Enlargement study) trial showed that patients with ejection fractions of < 40%, but no signs of heart failure, benefited from captopril treatment.

- Warfarin – if the patient has atrial fibrillation or has developed valvular problems (i.e. ruptured papillae), then they would benefit from anticoagulation therapy.

- Useful mnemonic:
  A   Aspirin
  B   Beta-blocker
  C   Cholesterol
  D   Diet
  E   Exercise

  ○ (2001) *Lancet*. **357**: 972–3.

Useful organisations

British Cardiac Society; www.bcs.com
Primary Care Cardiovascular Society; www.pccs.org.uk

Written question 12

> *You have been allocated a number of asylum seekers. A woman comes to see you with her son (who is translating) and her daughter (who appears to have learning disabilities). She is requesting HRT. How do you approach the consultation?*

Consultations involving language barriers and cultural issues are common in primary (and secondary) care. There are several issues raised here, and they cannot all be dealt with in one consultation.

Many asylum seekers will have telephone numbers for people who will translate for them over the telephone. This can be very useful, but brings into question the issue of confidentiality and real understanding. You will generally have no knowledge of the person who is translating.

Patient issues

- Why HRT?
  - Was the woman using HRT previously? If not, what has she read and why is she requesting it now?

- Menopause.
  - Is she menopausal or does she have symptoms that suggest she is perimenopausal? If this is the case, is it appropriate for her age?
  - What are her periods like?
  - Are there any risk factors for osteoporosis?
  - Does she need contraception?
  - Can she fully understand the risks vs. the benefits, given the method of translating?

- Other issues.
  - The psychological impact of status, a new country with higher costs of living, different cultures, etc.
  - Other medical/health promotion issues (e.g. chronic diseases and screening (cervical cytology), vaccinations, etc.).

Cultural issues

The fact that this woman's son is translating for her, especially when talking about gynaecological issues, may not be appropriate. Thus the information you think you are conveying and receiving in return may not be accurate.

Further family/social factors

- Are the woman's children now in school (given that they are new to the area)? Are they coping?

- Has her daughter had an educational needs assessment? Is she already on a Statement, given the impression you have (i.e. that of a learning disability)? Are there related medical issues that would need to be addressed?

- Is there any other adult support (e.g. father, family)?

- Is there an income?

- Understanding the circumstances behind a person seeking asylum leads to a better understanding, which can in turn improve their care. Certain problems, especially the psychological impact, can be pre-empted (to some extent) and addressed.

Doctor issues

- You need to be happy that the information you are receiving and trying to convey is accurate.

- Confidentiality – are you happy that translation is improving the care and understanding of this patient and not putting her at a disadvantage?

- Does she need contraceptive services or to be entered into the cervical screening programme?

- You have a duty of care to the children. New patients will need new patient checks to ensure that all of their needs are met to the best of your ability with the given resources.

Practice issues

- Is there an HRT protocol and leaflet? If not, is this an area to develop?

- Is there a new demand that would warrant translation of information/leaflets into another language?

- Is there a practice translator?

- What is the social services network like for those people who need further ongoing help?

The MRCGP oral examination

This may well be the most nerve-racking part of the exam. There is no anonymity as with the written paper, nor is editing allowed as with the video. This is you, warts and all.

The oral take place a few weeks after the written paper. For us this worked well, as we found that it was necessary to adopt a completely different approach. With our (made-up) questions we fired them blindly at each other only to find that we had to be quick thinking and professional, and that wisecracks didn't really work! We didn't think it was going too badly until we watched the RCGP video. This revealed that despite all our time in medicine we knew almost nothing about management, teambuilding, what qualities make a good chairperson, etc. We certainly didn't know the lingo to make ourselves sound convincing!

The oral exam is designed to determine how you will perform in real life (it is actually incredibly good practice for future interviews). It tests your communication skills, decision making and professional values in four main areas:

- care of patients
- working with colleagues
- the social role of general practice
- the doctor's personal responsibilities.

The exam consists of two consecutive 20-minute orals, each conducted by two examiners. There is a 5-minute break between the two parts, giving the examiners time to mark your performance. Each 20-minute exam will consist of approximately five questions.

Most of the time the examiners are pleasant and will try to help you if you are struggling or push you if you are doing well. Some people have reported a 'good cop, bad cop' style, but try not to be fazed if this happens.

One final tip – remember to dress smartly and polish your shoes!

We have put together 10 questions, again with thoughts on how you might approach the answers. We have used recent management and teambuilding books, etc., all of which are referenced at the end of the book (*see* page 271). Try to practise in pairs and make it like the exam. If an obvious question is raised from the answer, ask it, and if something is unclear, ask the person to explain it (that goes for the person asking the question as well as the one answering it). You don't have to talk willy-nilly for 5 minutes on each question. If you reach a natural pause, that is fine – the examiner will then ask you something else.

Oral question 1

A patient you have been treating is now in the end stages of heart failure. He cannot wash himself without becoming extremely short of breath. If he were to ask you to help him end things quickly and peacefully, how would you respond?

This is obviously a question on euthanasia, which is still a crime in the UK.

There are a number of issues.

Quality of life

Presumably for this patient it is poor. It is important to find out what is the worst thing for him (e.g. lack of dignity, feeling unwell, etc.).

- Listen to and empathise with his concerns and health beliefs.

- Anything you offer him should be aimed at improving the quality of the life he has left.

Medical treatment options

These are aimed at maximising heart failure treatment. Any unnecessary treatment should be stopped.

- Diuretics (e.g. could his renal function tolerate metolazone?).

- Nitrates/ACE inhibitors.

- Beta-blockers are unlikely to be warranted at this stage, but are worth considering.

- Home oxygen.

- Morphine, diazepam, etc. in small doses are often very helpful.
- Is the patient becoming clinically depressed? Does this need treatment?
- Does he need an acute admission?

Primary healthcare team

- Occupational therapists, district nurses and social services should all be involved, with the patient's consent. The community psychiatric nurse may also be of benefit.
- In some areas, if there are beds available, a hospice may take such patients for respite or palliative care.
- Teamwork and good communication are fundamental to successful care. Remember that the most important member of the team is the patient.

Euthanasia

However much you may empathise with your patient, euthanasia would be viewed in a legal context as murder. Patients usually understand this and do not pressure their doctors further.

Advance directives

Is it an appropriate time to discuss eventualities (e.g. in the event of a cardiac arrest). To arrange an advance directive, the patient would need legal council and have to be fully informed of all possible eventualities.

Cultural issues

- What religion is your patient? Would he appreciate input from the local church/ mosque, etc.?
- Is part of the reason he is requesting euthanasia because of personal/cultural beliefs about cleanliness and nursing?

The examiners, if you have not already answered, may push you on whether or not you would help this man to die. Given the legal implications, whatever your view it would be prudent to answer 'no' – possibly adding that you would help to keep him as comfortable as possible with the appropriate support.

This question could easily apply to patients with cancer, multiple sclerosis, motor neuron disease (recent high-profile court case), etc., and it will be topical for some time yet.

It is important to show that you empathise with the patient and will do your best to maximise the quality of time he has left, but that you also understand the legal boundaries.

Oral question 2

What do you understand by the term 'medical ethics'?

Ethical reasoning is a branch of philosophy that deals with right and wrong. In the UK law is either statute (acts passed by Parliament) or common (law formed on precedent and judicial interpretation of statute).

GPs need to be aware of both legal and ethical frameworks on medical issues.

The four model principle

This allows analysis of a problem, but not necessarily its resolution.

1 Beneficence – the principle that doctors should only do good for their patients.

2 Non-maleficence – the principle that a doctor should do no harm.

3 Justice – the principle that scarce healthcare resources should be shared fairly. This is distributive rather than criminal justice.

4 Autonomy – the principle that all patients should have the right of self-determi-nation. A fully autonomous decision should be informed, competent and not coerced.

The four moral theory

1 Theory of virtue – describes innate character attributes that are either good or bad.

2 Theory of duties – rationally based rules of moral conduct. In the UK, these rules are set out as GMC regulations.

3 Theory of utility – describes what is morally good in terms of the 'greatest good for the greatest number'.

4 Theory of rights – describes social relationships between people such that some have an obligation to provide a service to others based on intrinsic right.

If you cite one ethical model and show that you understand it, you will have done well. The obvious follow-on question is 'Do you know any other ethical models?'. If you don't, say that you do not know them well enough to explain them, you have found a model that works for you, and that this is generally what you try to apply to help you to analyse a situation (or something along those lines!). If you can remember other models, then certainly describe them.

Oral question 3

Do you think prescribing rationale has changed over the last 40 years?

- All of the evidence suggests that the answer to this question is yes.
- The availability of drugs has increased (different drug classes as well as drugs with the same class effect).
- We have an ageing society with the associated diseases and problems. This will often mean multiple drug regimes to improve morbidity, mortality and quality of life. The average elderly person now has 8.8 items on repeat prescription.
- We as doctors are more aware of evidence-based prescribing issues, as well as the fact that there is more research on the safety profile of a given drug.
- Much of our work is now about primary prevention (e.g. coronary heart disease risk and the use of statins).
- There has been an increase in different types of advertising of drugs available on prescription and over the counter. This increases patient awareness (a good thing), but it also increases the financial burden on the NHS (a bad thing, especially when a patient is requesting a drug that is not warranted).
- Even in the absence of advertising, patient awareness and demand are increasing as information becomes increasingly accessible on the Internet.
- GPs are now prescribing and monitoring drugs that were previously only available in secondary care (e.g. fertility drugs). This obviously impacts on a GP's drug budget and medicolegal pitfalls about prescribing specialist drugs.
- Our knowledge of antibiotic resistance is increasing, and GPs have altered their prescribing habits accordingly. Another example of changing prescribing habits would be blood pressure control.
- External factors that impact on GP prescribing include the following:
  - personal experience
  - National Service Frameworks and NICE
  - local primary care group and primary care trust guidance
  - local consultant preferences – as patients are discharged on certain drugs
  - patient pressure
  - pharmacological companies (representatives, drug deals for dispensing practices)
  - local educational meetings and guest speakers.

This question would lead nicely on to others such as the following:

Do you think nurse prescribing will impact on GP prescribing budgets/PACT data?

Do you think nurse prescribing will undo the hard work of public health and GPs in encouraging self-management of minor ailments and the reductions achieved in anti-biotic prescribing?

How would you go about implementing nurse prescribing in your practice?

All of these question raise issues such as the following:

- whether nurses want to expand their role (the first question to answer)
- training issues
- the drawing up of protocols and patient group directives
- supervision and accessibility of GPs
- audit
- the issue of nurse practitioners having their own lists, especially in inner-city areas where there is often difficulty in recruiting GPs.

The Royal College of General Practitioners is in favour of nurse prescribing by nurses who wish to develop these skills, but recognises the need for training and support. There must be safeguards for nurses with revalidation.

The CROWN Review recommended the following:

- a period of supervised practice
- drugs to which 'new prescribers' have access would be subject to expert clinical pharmacology and safety vetting
- the need for training and education.

○ (1999) Extended prescribing: nurse prescribing and the CROWN Review. *Hosp Med.* **60**: 718–21.

Oral question 4

How do you think flexible training and employment will affect general practice?

This does not have to apply to doctors, but can include nursing, reception and office staff, depending on how you want to frame your answer.

Currently more than 50% of medical-school intake is female. Women represent over 30% of the GP workforce, and the numbers appear to be increasing. Although it is not solely a female issue (other than the need for maternity leave!), family life and childcare impact greatly on the need for work to be flexible in order to get the most from employees.

Advantages

- Flexible training and employment allow flexible career choices.
- They make a profession more appealing because of that flexibility.

- They improve personal fulfilment (e.g. the decision with regard to quality vs. income).

- GPs and medically trained professionals may be encouraged to stay in the profession (i.e. work can fit in with family life).

- Cynically, it means that the NHS gets more for its money, as part-time workers will virtually always work more than the hours for which they are paid and although people who work full-time do too, there are more hours on to which the work can encroach if you are part time.

- Flexible working can improve time management and organisation, as it is less easy to put things off until tomorrow.

- It will hopefully reduce stress, burnout and the number of people who retire early.

- It may reduce the amount of sick leave taken.

- It may reduce the number of people who would have to retrain because they had taken time out to raise a family.

- It would increase the number of people employed, and so decrease unemployment and benefits claimed (thinking in terms of office and reception staff).

Disadvantages

- If people work part-time, there will need to be even more doctors and staff.

- The overall cost for the NHS will increase (training, pay, National Insurance, superannuation, sick pay, maternity pay, etc.).

- Access for patients may become an issue, especially if a practice works on the principle that doctors see their own registered patients. This would obviously disadvantage the patients of the doctor who is working part-time.

- There may be less job satisfaction (e.g. if you are caring for a palliative care patient and they need care when you are not available, this may affect continuity of care and treatment success).

- There may be practice issues (hence the value of a well-considered practice agreement detailing even the smallest points on the distribution of workload) where a full-time partner feels that a part-time partner ought to put in more time, or is even jealous because they cannot go part-time.

- You may not be at work when certain meetings take place. This raises the need for agendas and good minute keeping and circulation.

Oral question 5

Do you think disease registers have a place in modern-day healthcare?

The answer to this question is yes, particularly for chronic disease management. However, disease registers raise numerous issues for patients, doctors, nurses and administration staff.

Advantages

- Disease registers help to target patient groups (e.g. diabetics, asthmatics, coronary heart disease, etc.) to ensure that they are receiving the best care.
- It is easier to:
  - audit management success against set criteria
  - recall patients for follow-up
  - communicate with secondary care and the primary care group/primary care trust.
- It may mean that patients receive better care (although this is not a foregone conclusion):
  - guidelines are developed consistent with available evidence
  - clinics focus on specific problems (so these are not just glossed over when consulting for a sore throat).
- Disease registers may be linked to pay and future funding (this is also a disadvantage in some cases).
- Although initially the process will be time consuming (especially the hours needed to complete the register), once complete it should be relatively simple to update.

Disadvantages

- Doctors and nurses may become so preoccupied with ticking boxes that they forget the patient.
- Templates and keeping the register up to date can be time consuming if they are not simple.
- Disease registers do not assess quality.
- There are consent and confidentiality issues for the patients (by virtue of their being on a register).
- It is necessary to ensure that all doctors and nurses are completing the relevant areas (i.e. that there is continued motivation).
- If a practice is not computerised/computer-literate, this is an arduous task. Although part of the NHS plan is that all practices should be computerised,

this does not necessarily mean that all practices will make good use of those systems.

- If you have patients who are non-compliant and uninterested (e.g. in their HbA_{1C} levels), and who have not reached the point where they wish to be 'educated', then they may affect your figures, which may in turn affect your pay. There needs to be some way to take into account compliance, depending on what you want to achieve with your register.

Oral question 6

What do you understand by quality within the NHS?

Quality is all about standards – and being able to give people (patients and staff) what they need as well as what they want. It does this at the lowest possible cost (i.e. is economical).
    It includes the following:

- development:
    - of staff and the organisation
    - of new methods

- objective measurements:
    - audit
    - quarterly statistics
    - satisfaction questionnaires, etc.

- productivity:
    - improved satisfaction that is economical.

Or, alternatively:

- patient quality:
    - what do they want from the service?

- professional quality:
    - education and training issues
    - revalidation

- management quality:
    - helps to ensure efficient, productive use of resources available.

Clinical governance should feature somewhere in your discussion about controlling quality.
    This question could lead on to the following one:

Why is quality important?

- It improves satisfaction all around (among patients/clients and staff).

- Work is more enjoyable and less frustrating.

- It increases productivity and control.

- It reduces unnecessary costs, and this increases potential income.

- It reduces the likelihood of complaints and negligence claims.

- It improves staff morale and interprofessional co-operation.

- It makes recruitment and retention easier in a competitive labour market.

- It avoids duplication (e.g. of administrative tasks).

- It enhances reputation, which is good for morale and business in a competitive market.

- It creates a focus for development strategies – a service cannot be 'all things to all people', so it is important to single out groups of people for a particular service.

What sort of issues would you look at when determining quality features?

- Competence:
  - of employees
  - appropriate skills and training to perform as you would expect.

- Communication:
  - with clients
  - not just in a consultation context, but also ways to keep them informed of changes and listen to their concerns.

- Credibility:
  - honesty towards staff and patients.

- Security:
  - physical safety, confidentiality, etc.

- Courtesy:
  - client orientation of staff
  - polite, friendly staff with the ability to listen.

- Access:
  - a service needs to be readily accessible.

- Reliability:
  - this ties in with credibility.

- Physical tangibles:
  - the environment and appearance of the staff reflect the people who work there and their employers.

Oral question 7

As a GP, how would you facilitate good methods of communication between staff?

Effective communication is essential if a team is to be successful. It saves time and reduces unnecessary frustrations.

There are different methods of communication:

- message books/notes
- computer
- meetings with minutes that are subsequently distributed or displayed
- appraisals
- a complaints procedure.

Whatever method is used for a particular issue needs to be reliable, and will work better if it is agreed by all users.

Part of making communication effective is creating a dynamic team. This involves leadership skills and getting to know people.

Three key factors are common to all effective teams:

1 identification of roles so that there is no confusion

2 having effective and efficient processes in place

3 maintaining a high level of morale.

Building and evolving that team involves the following:

- honesty about current effectiveness
- tackling problems (including personality clashes) head on and working through them
- being prepared to learn new skills as a group.

   You mentioned meetings as a method of communication. What do you think distinguishes a good meeting from a not-so-good one?

Meetings need to have a purpose and a conclusion. There needs to be consideration as to timing, objectives, venue and the individuals who should be included. Meetings need to occur regularly, and there also needs to be an effective chair with good facilitation.

John Cleese's *Meetings, Bloody Meetings* gives a short sensible guide to successful meetings.

1 Plan ahead – what is the meeting for?

2 Prenotification – agenda.

3 Preparation – agenda, order of priority and a guide to time available.

4 Processing
   - each discussion needs structure
   - the chairperson must understand the group dynamics to help to ensure that conflict is creative rather than destructive.

5 Putting it on record
   - summary of events, decisions made and actions to be taken.

Another frame is 'The Four Ds' from *The PCG Team Builder*.

- Define the problem.

- Define the objective in looking for a solution (consensus/vote/delegate to certain members).

- Decide how to effect a successful solution.

- Determine how you will measure success (evaluate ideas against value/benefit, cost, feasibility, and the resources available).

Tell me more about the chairperson. What do you understand their role to be?

The chairperson's role is to provide a framework, to maintain the focus and to facilitate – getting the best from all members of the team, as well as getting people to work together as a team.

1 Framework:
   - maintain organisation and time-keeping
   - identify when things are drifting/going awry
   - generate options to stop people becoming blinkered
   - set standards (firm but fair).

2 Focus on the issue at hand:
   - clarify points, summarise
   - deal with time-wasting.

3 Facilitation:
   - allow flexibility and freedom for expression of views
   - understand others and listen to them
   - remain unbiased and neutral/impartial
   - encourage co-operation
   - recognise that it is a team effort, and that the chairperson cannot make the team effective on their own
   - be sensitive and respectful.

4 Another summary:
   – communicate
   – control
   – co-ordinate
   – coax
   – compare
   – clarify
   – concentrate.

Oral question 8

What qualities should a modern GP have?

See the General Medical Council's *Duties of a Doctor*.

- They should:
  – be clinically competent
  – be the patient's advocate
  – be a good team player
  – have or develop leadership skills
  – be a partner or business person
  – be a reflective practitioner, with self-awareness
  – be open to new ideas, flexible and tolerant
  – be a good teacher
  – be a gatekeeper and resource allocater
  – not be prejudiced
  – avoid discrimination
  – be aware of how their personal beliefs may affect the care that they give/offer
  – treat information with respect, and maintain confidentiality
  – be involved in personal and professional growth (revalidation)
  – be able to recognise stresses and hopefully adapt in order to prevent burnout in themselves, colleagues and employees.

- They should have an ethical and cultural awareness as well as moral principles.

- They may be an employer (or a representative of one) and all that this implies (listener, facilitator, fair, enthusiastic, diplomatic).

- They should have an understanding of medicolegal issues.

- They may be involved in research, and should always be involved in audit.

- They should be prepared to talk around all of the above issues.

- The European branch of the World Organisation of Family Doctors (WONCA) has developed a new definition of general practice, which is not too disimilar to the GMC's *Duties of a Doctor*.

Oral question 9

How would you inform a patient that they have ovarian cancer following the results of investigations you have ordered?

This is a question about good communication skills and the breaking of bad news.

- Have all the facts available, and double-check that they are for the correct person.
- Establish that the patient wants to know more.
- Establish what they already understand.
- Choose the right moment. You will need time, privacy and quiet (i.e. no disturbances). Consider whether a relative should be present.
- Keep checking that you are giving the right amount of information and that it is wanted.
- Ask the patient what their main concerns are.
- Find out how they are feeling.
- Do not rush on to treatment. When they are ready, outline a management plan.
- Ensure that there is adequate follow-up and support.
- Throughout, acknowledge the patient's feelings, distress, etc.
- Recognise that there will be psychological, social, spiritual and cultural aspects.
- Always try and communicate with the practice team so that everyone is aware of the situation.
- Housekeeping (Neighbour's gem).
- Acknowledge your own feelings.

If the patient has little awareness, how would you convey the news without pushing them into denial or provoking overwhelming distress?

- Fire a warning shot (e.g. 'I'm afraid I have bad news').
- Try to give them time, so that they ask for the information rather than you forcing the issue.
- Use silence.

If the patient's relatives asked you not to give the diagnosis to the patient, what would you do?

This raises issues of confidentiality.

You should ask yourself why you were talking to the relatives rather than the patient in the first place.

There is no right answer here – it depends on the situation.

Be aware that advances in oncology and surgery have resulted in improved morbidity and mortality in many cancers. Not divulging the information denies the patient these treatments as well as denying palliative care with the Macmillan nurses when the time comes.

Oral question 10

How would you go about negotiating a change in working patterns (for example) within your practice?

There are various strategies that may encourage people to think about change and take action towards making that change. If people are involved, they are likely to accept and contribute to change.

The responses that people may have to change are variable.

- Some ignore it.
- Some resist it.
- Some go along with it passively.
- Some plan ahead.
- Some grasp the opportunity and actively pursue it.

There are five main qualities needed to effect successful change:

- enthusiasm
- energy
- determination
- diplomacy
- foresight.

A simple model for change

1 Where are you now?
   - Motives (financial, psychological, status, reputation, achievement, creativity).
   - Priorities.
   - Talents in relation to change.
   - Time allocation.
2 Where do you want to get to?
   - Define your aims, set goals and promote ownership.
   - Agree priorities.
   - Define criteria for success and failure.
   - Define a time scale.

3 How are you going to get there?
- Clarify resources.
- Clarify obstructions and helpful factors.
- Conduct a SWOT analysis (strengths, weaknesses, opportunities and threats).
- Select a team and 'create' time for that team.

Domain mapping (Spiegal et al.)

This is quite a useful technique which can encourage all parties with an interest to contribute to an analysis of the effects of any proposed change.

1 Draw six concentric circles.

2 Divide them into as many segments as there are interested parties/stakeholders.

3 Enter the details:
- proposed change
- name of the stakeholder
- current involvement in the situation where change is proposed
- future benefits of the change for each person
- potential costs to each person of the proposed change
- potential power of stakeholders to obstruct change.

You may be pushed to say how you would make those changes (i.e. implement them).

- Involve the relevant people.

- Be thorough in your considerations, and don't just change for the sake of it.

- Make clear concise plans. As with guidelines, involving people creates ownership.

- Have a time scale – be realistic and flexible.

- Have a measure of success/failure (e.g. audit, observation, etc.)

Video: summative assessment/MRCGP single route

The single route is by far the most efficient way of doing the consultation skills, but you have to be organised to get it all completed to the correct standard. You *must* familiarise yourself fully with the exam criteria (www.rcgp.org.uk) early in the game. The summative assessment handbook is available from the National Office for Summative Assessment at www.nosa.org.uk.

Seven consultations are required for the MRCGP (these should be the first seven on the tape). Recordings for the summative assessment need to be 2 hours long, with no less than eight consultations (you really should do this just in case you fail the MRCGP).

The *MRCGP Video Workbook* contains the following:

- the competencies to be demonstrated (performance criteria):
  - discover the reason for the patient's attendance
  - define the clinical problem(s)
  - explain the problem(s) to the patient
  - address the patient's problem(s)
  - make effective use of the consultation

- detailed instructions for recording consultations

- a video log

- consultation summary forms

- ethical principles.

There is not a great deal of additional direction needed for the video. Working for the rest of the exam will automatically improve your knowledge and performance on tape. You need to start recording early and get used to taping yourself. If you are uncomfortable, not only will the patient sense this, but you will start to make unnecessary mistakes. Using the tapes to identify your learning needs represents good use of your time.

The taping itself is the easy part. You then have to sit down and go through the tapes with the performance criteria to hand. You need to give this your whole attention, as it is the only way to find out what points you miss.

Involving your trainer (if you are still a registrar) or colleagues is very important. They have a great deal of experience and will help you to identify your unidentified gaps. Discuss how they prefer to view your tapes. Unless you want to demonstrate a specific point, it can become a monumental waste of time to go through the tapes you already know are unlikely to pass. Your trainer will probably thank you for editing these out and getting straight to the ones that you think may be good enough.

It is important to remember that the tape needs to be at normal speed (short play), the time needs to be visible (on a clock or screen) and you must have the consent forms. Leave yourself plenty of time to edit on to VHS and complete the workbook.

It is worth noting that, depending on your circumstances, you may be able to apply to do the simulated patients instead of the video component. This is one session and, rather like the oral, there is no editing!

Membership by assessment and performance (MAP)

This is a relatively new route to gaining membership. It is geared towards GPs who have been in practice for more than 5 years and are able to demonstrate the quality of care that they provide.

You can purchase the MAP handbook from the Royal College of General

Practitioners. This sets out the criteria, which are divided into three broad groupings, namely *You and Your Practice*, *Managing Illness*, and *Learning and Values*.
   MAP consists of three separate elements:

- a video assessment or simulated surgery

- a portfolio of written evidence (up to nine submissions)

- a practice visit.

Relatively few candidates choose this route, but among those who have passed and written about their experience it seems as if the general feelings are similar – it is hard work, but the rewards are great for practice, patient and doctor.

Examinations and courses to consider

Summative assessment

Audit

This is probably the one part of the summative assessment that, in theory, you can do in your hospital posts, so long as the topic audited is relevant to general practice.

- The information on what is expected and how to present the work can be obtained from the Region or from your course organisers.

- If you do leave it until your registrar year, remember that you have to complete the audit cycle to show that changes have been successfully implemented.

- The message is to keep it simple and start early (within the first 2 months). Write it up at the time when you do the audit, while it is fresh in your mind.

Multiple-choice questions (MCQs)

- It is not recommended that you take this part of the exam until you have spent at least 3 months in practice. This is because of the management issues that you will not have encountered in hospital.

- Some candidates use this exam as a mock for the MRCGP, to identify the gaps in their knowledge.

- However, if you do the MRCGP MCQs prior to taking the summative assessment, then you do not need to take the summative assessment MCQ paper.

Video

- Again the key is to start early – the task will be loathsome unless you warm to it!

- Use the early tapes to improve your consulting style. Be objective and ask for your trainer's opinion.

- Read all of the information, especially the marking scheme.

- It is important that the sessions in which you decide to video run smoothly. You do not want a perfect consultation to be sabotaged at the end with a discussion about the consent form and where to sign.

- Ask the receptionists to inform patients that you are videoing and to request them to sign the consent form in reception (before and after the consultation).

- If possible, give yourself longer appointments on the days when you are videoing.

Trainer's report

This does not need to be formally completed until the end of your registrar year. Read it at the beginning. There are some areas in which your trainer has to be sure that you are competent. This may mean watching you perform certain tasks.

If possible, try to complete the report as you go along.

You can obtain the information for each part of the exam from your course organisers, the region, or JCPTGP, 14 Princes Gate, Hyde Park, London SW7 1PU (tel. 0207 581 3232). This will be superseded by the Postgraduate Medical Education and Training Board (PMETB).

The UKCRA have published a booklet entitled *Summative Assessment GP Training*. If you have not received it, it is available from the National Office for Summative Assessment, NHS Executive South & West, Highcroft, Romsey Road, Winchester SO22 5DH.

While going through your hospital posts

Remember to get all of your VTR/2 forms signed and stamped at the end of each of your jobs. Do this as you go along, as trying to find consultants (and getting them to remember you) two years down the line can be incredibly frustrating. These forms are kept either by your VTS secretary or by medical staffing. They are the proof you need to obtain your final certificate.

Diplomas to Consider

DRCOG (Diploma of the Royal College of Obstetricians and Gynaecologists)
This is not necessary for general practice, but if you look at job advertisements, some practices stipulate that they would like applicants to have the diploma. You can only do this exam (by MCQs and OSCE) after at least 3 months of obstetrics and gynaecology.

If you want to attempt it, request the information from the college early on.

Royal College of Obstetricians and Gynaecologists, 27 Sussex Place, Regent's Park, London NW1 4RG.
Tel. 020 7772 6200.
www.rcog.org.uk

DFFP (Diploma of the Faculty of Family Planning)

This again is not essential for general practice unless you want to do family planning sessions or fit coils. You can do ad hoc family planning sessions (earning the equivalent of £30 or more/hour) once you have the diploma, while you are still doing either hospital posts or your GP registrar year.

Once you have done the DFFP, you can then do the coil training for the IUD letters of competence (up to five coils in the DFFP training can count towards the 10 that are needed) and the implant training.

If you are considering doing this diploma, you will need to have completed a minimum of 3 months obstetrics and gynaecology (you can do the theory before this, which is a 3.5-day course if it includes the coil information).

The syllabus and logbook can be viewed on the faculty website:
www.ffprhc.org.uk (under general training committee).

Faculty of Family Planning and Reproductive Health, 19 Cornwall Terrace, London NW1 4QP.
Tel. 020 7724 5647.

DCH (Diploma in Child Health)

This is a detailed diploma involving practical-based sessions as well as the exam. It may be possible to do these sessions through your paediatric job.

Only a few places seem to be requesting this diploma but, as is often the case, it may be something that tips the balance in your favour.

Royal College of Paediatrics and Child Health,
50 Hallam Street, London W1 6DE.
Tel. 020 7307 5600
www.rcpch.ac.uk/

Courses to consider through hospital posts

During your GP registrar year your study leave budget is around £200 (unless your VTS has some extra to use up), whereas in hospital posts it is around £500. Double-check these figures for your trust. Use the study leave time and money wisely, bearing in mind that if you want to go on revision courses this will use a lot of your registrar allocation.

Advanced life support (ALS)

Ensure that this is up to date before your registrar year, and that you have a signed form confirming that you are qualified in ALS. If you are thinking of taking the

MRCGP, you need to have basic life support, which the ALS training incorporates. Most trusts provide this training free of charge for trust employees.

Acupuncture

Many hospital trusts will fund acupuncture courses. Acupuncture is as relevant to general practice as you want to make it. The courses tend to be held at weekends, which means that getting the study leave is not part of the ordeal. A good basic course to ensure that you are competent to practise would take about 4 days.

Information can be found in the *British Medical Journal* advertisements. See also:

British Medical Acupuncture Society (BMAS), Newton House, Newton Lane, Whitley, Warrington WA4 4JA.
Tel. 01925 730727.
www.medical-acupuncture.co.uk

Some half-day release courses (or within your postgraduate region) will offer the following courses to GP registrars:

- alternative medicine

- ENT

- ophthalmology

- dermatology

- general practice management issues

- communication skills.

All of the above, and more, would be time well spent. It is all about developing your own interests and deciding what type of service you would like to be able to offer your patients. For example, acupuncture can be done safely during a 10-minute consultation and can give incredible relief (a popular misconception is that you need a good half hour).

Courses to consider during your registrar year

Minor surgery

You can pay to go on a minor surgery course while doing your hospital training. GP registrars can usually go on the course without having to pay.

If you want to be signed up by your primary care trust for minor surgery so that you can claim payment for it, then it is necessary to arrange this.

The theoretical course is *not* the way in which you will become competent in minor surgery. You will learn this either through your trainer or through other colleagues (e.g. dermatologists, surgeons, rheumatologists, etc.).

Child health surveillance
Again this is necessary if you want to do child health surveillance (i.e. baby checks) and claim payment for it.

The course is usually 'free' for GP registrars if done in your region. You can pay to do it earlier in your training.

Palliative care
Most regions are now running palliative care courses, again with no payment being required for GP registrars.

Although palliative care is unlikely to be a huge part of day-to-day life, it will be the one thing that, if you do it well, you will be remembered for.

The course teaches the knowledge base as well as the practical issues (e.g. how to set up a syringe driver).

Check list

Course/Exam		Date completed
Family planning (DFFP)	Theory Practical IUD	
DRCOG	Course (?) Exam	
Advanced life support		
DCH		
Child health surveillance		
Minor surgery		
Palliative care		
Summative assessment	Audit MCQ Video Trainer's report	
MRCGP	MCQ Written Oral Video/simulated patients	
Others		

Publications to subscribe to

You should already be receiving the Chief Medical Officer's Updates, the *Drug and Therapeutics Bulletin*, etc.

Update   www.DoctorUpdate.net
                                Tel. 020 8652 8454 (circulation enquiries)

The Practitioner   CMP Information Ltd, Ludgate House, 245 Blackfriars Road, London SE1 9UR.
                                Tel. 020 7921 8120

GP (newspaper)   174 Hammersmith Road, London W6 7JP.
                                www.GPonline.com
                                This is also the contact for *Medeconomics* (they also issue *MIMS*)

Pulse (newspaper)   CMP Information Ltd, Ludgate House, 245 Blackfriars Road, London SE1 9UR.
                                Tel. 020 7921 8120

Health and Ageing   Medicom(UK) Ltd, Churston House, Portsmouth Road, Esher, Surrey KT10 9AD.
                                Tel. 01372 471671

Geriatric Medicine   Medpress (a division of Inside Communications Media Ltd), Isis Building, Thames Key, 193 Marsh Wall, London E14 9SG.
                                Tel. 020 7772 8300

GP registrar money issues

Salary

This is paid by the practice (which is reimbursed by the primary care trust). It includes the car allowance.

Mileage

Mileage for visits can be claimed back from the primary care trust. This does not include mileage to work (unless there is a visit on the way).

Mileage for visits is also tax-deductible. If you fill in a tax return you will have to declare the money you are reimbursed.

Defence union

This is reimbursed by the primary care trust. Usually the practice manager claims this back for you.

Relocation allowance and telephone rental and installation

Expenses which will probably be tax-deductible

- *Professional subscriptions*: GMC, *BMJ*, DRCOG, DFFP, Defence Union, etc.
- *Mileage*: for visits, not to and from work; if you are working as a locum, all mileage is tax-deductible because you are working from home.
- *Office at home*: running costs, rates, electricity and gas are worked out as a proportion depending on the number of rooms in your house/square footage.
- *Computer*: if you use it for work.
- *Stationery*: used for work (e.g. paper, envelopes, stamps/postage, acetates).
- *MRCGP*: this is necessary if you want to be involved in training.
- *Courses*: if you pay for them (if you are reimbursed you must declare this).
- *Telephone expenses*: if you are using your home telephone for work, then ensure that you obtain an itemised bill so that you are able to calculate the correct amount.
- *VTS*: the videos for summative assessment and the MRCGP; you are unlikely to be able to justify the purchase of video equipment, as this should be supplied by your training practice; Internet links from home.
- *Miscellaneous*: digital camera if used for work purposes/teaching/publications (if it is also used at home, then a proportion of the cost is calculated); books and equipment if these are necessary for your job.

Keep up-to-date records (ideally a spreadsheet) of all income and expenses.

Speak to the business advisers at the Inland Revenue, as you are self-employed as a GP. They are an excellent source of information, and will help you with your tax return if necessary. It is prudent to remember who they work for!

Remember that you will have to declare all incoming monies (e.g. cremation fees, DS 1500s, etc.). Even if you have not filled in a tax return while doing your hospital jobs, you could still be investigated, and this is especially likely if your first tax return is as a GP. Get used to doing them early when the figures are easier!

Always keep all of your receipts.

Self-employment as a GP/locum

This follows on from the registrar issues. Good records are essential. Outgoings that are tax-deductible are similar.

Because GPs provide a service (rather than receiving a contract of service as in other NHS professions), we have a self-employed, independent contractor status.

Once you have qualified as a GP, you need to register yourself as being self-employed with the Inland Revenue. If you do not register within 3 months of starting work, you will probably be fined.

You will find some information as well as a selection of relevant publications at www.inlandrevenue.gov.uk.

Helpline for the newly self-employed: 08459 15 45 15

This is to register. Alternatively, you can complete a form CWF1.

By registering as self-employed you will pay Class 2 National Insurance (NI) contributions. At the end of the tax year, when you send in your self-assessment, the amount of NI contributions you owe will be calculated. This is then payable as Class 4 NI at the same time as you pay your income-tax bill.

You also need to ensure that you are registered with a primary care trust on their supplementary list.

Locum jobs

- Negotiate pay before doing a job. Ask around and find out what other people are charging.

- Negotiate what work is to be done (length of surgery, number of appointments, visits, etc.).

- Once the job is complete, or on a weekly/monthly basis, invoice the practice.
  - If you do not do this, you are unlikely to get paid.
  - If you take the invoice with you on the final day, it saves on postage.

- Locums can now contribute to the superannuation scheme. Your primary care trust will have the relevant information. If you ask them, they will send you the forms that you will need the practice to complete to prove what your earnings have been.

  Information is also available from the NHS Pensions Agency: Tel. 01253 774774; www.NHSPA.gov.uk.

- Try to save around 40% of your income in a high-interest account for payment of the following:
  - income tax
  - Class 4 National Insurance
  - superannuation
  - Defence Union subscriptions for next year.

Considerations when looking for a GP post

- Full-time or part-time.

- PMS or GMS practice.

- Salaried, partnership or retainer.

- Portfolio career option.

- Outside work you may want to do:
  - clinical assistant post
  - family planning
  - private health screening
  - obesity clinics
  - local medical committee
  - primary care group/primary care trust, etc.
  - post-marketing surveillance work
  - forensic work.

- If you are considering a partnership:
  - rural/inner-city location
  - where in the country
  - how many partners
  - how many sessions you want to work
  - whether you want to be involved in training or with medical students
  - whether you want a dispensing practice
  - how involved you want to be in antenatal care, child health surveillance, minor surgery, etc.
  - whether other members of the primary healthcare team have a base at the practice
  - what computer system is used
  - who does the auditing
  - what role the practice nurses have (nurse practitioner?)
  - what the premises are like
  - what car parking is like (small things can become very irritating)
  - how the appraisals work and who does them
  - what the local hospitals, educational meetings and outpatient waiting times are like
  - what security is like
  - what meetings take place (weekly business, nurse, practice, in-house educational, etc.).

- Does the practice hold social events?

- Other issues:
  - what are the local schools (comprehensive and public) like?
  - what are house prices like in the area?
  - what are the road/motorway links like?

These are just some things to consider – the list is not exhaustive. Work out where you are coming from, and do not rush into anything. Locum work can be lucrative, despite the fact that you do not get holiday pay!

Partnership agreement

If you are a member of the BMA, request a copy of *Medical Partnership under the NHS*. This should get you orientated with regard to what issues a practice agreement should cover. You should be thinking about signing a written mutual agreement at the end of your period of mutual assessment. It is foolhardy to enter into a partnership with no written agreement in place. In such an instance this is a partnership at will, which can be brought to an end as quickly as it is formed.

It is advisable to take specialist independent legal (and accountancy) advice before signing. You need to protect yourself, no matter how well you think you know your partners.

What should it cover?

1   All parties' names and addresses.

2   Commencement date.

3   Declaration relating to termination of partnership, retirement, a party wishing to move, gross misconduct, etc.

4   Capital assets:
    – sale and purchasing of shares
    – valuation methods, especially in relation to cost rent scheme.

5   Occupation of premises by non-owning partners.

6   Expenses – individual and partnership.

7   Income – individual and partnership, especially notional/cost rent income and outside work (to be pooled?).

8   Schedule of profit shares from commencement date to parity.

9   Partners' obligations to each other.

10   Partnership accounts (drawings, tax reserve, year end, accountants).

11   Superannuation.

12   Holiday and study leave.

13   Sickness, maternity and paternity entitlement.

14   Effect of retirement or death – restrictive covenant.

15   Arbitration of provisions.

16   Declaration about patients.

Things to consider in detail prior to accepting

Negotiate terms (this will involve compromise).

Commitment to the practice

- Sessions to be worked.
- Outside interests/work (pool the earnings?).

Finances

- Determine cost of buying in time to parity.
- Profit shares.

Voting rights

Some matters should only be acted upon with unanimous agreement (e.g. appointment of a new partner).

- One vote per partner is ideal.
- Part-time partners should have equal voting power if they buy into a share of the profits, but are 'jointly' liable and have the same professional interest in the business.

Maternity leave

- Currently 18 weeks (soon to be increased), it can be claimed to cover locum costs.
- Time allowed must be fair.
- Determine what will happen to drawings and who will cover the locum costs.
- Paternity leave details are equally important.

Expulsion clauses (e.g. lengthy incapacity, gross misconduct).

Expenses (this includes everything, e.g. phones, subscriptions, courses and travel, equipment, books, etc.). What will be covered by the practice; what will be paid for personally?

Accounts

When considering buying into a practice, one thing it is necessary to look over and understand (to a certain degree) is the practice accounts.

We are not accountants, and certainly we make no claim to be experts on the subject. Going through the process and having to put your name to the yearly accounts makes you learn quickly. We hope that you will find this Noddy-like guide a useful starting point.

In short, you are looking at four issues.

- Is the practice solvent?

- How much will you be drawing?

- Have there been any major changes from one year to the next, and if so, why?

- Where could the practice potentially improve?

When you receive the accounts they will probably be in a summarised format (i.e. they will not include every single transaction, but will have sections grouped together).

Look at the year of the accounts that you are given. Some run from 6 April to 5 April (i.e. the tax year), while others run from 1 January to 31 December. It really does not matter, but do be aware that you may be looking at accounts which are well over 12 months old.

In the accounts you should see two columns of figures – the current year and the previous year for easy comparison.

Look at each of the following.

- The layout.
  - Is it a logical format?
  - Is it clear where the numbers are from? If not, ask.

- How were the figures calculated?

- How did performance compare with previous years?
  - How does it compare with the national average (often represented graphically at the end of the accounts using information from Medeconomics)?
  - What areas can be improved?

- Are the following shown clearly?
  - Value and ownership of property.
  - Fixed assets (fixtures, fittings, computers, furniture, drug stock).
  - Investments and running costs.

- Are postgraduate education allowance, seniority pay, etc. kept personally or pooled?

- Does the practice pay for GMC, Defence Union and professional subscriptions, etc.?

- How much profit was made? And was this shared fairly in line with the partner-ship agreement?

- Is there a partnership tax account?

- How much tax and National Insurance are you likely to pay?

- Is there an accountant's report (a summary of the important features of the accounts)?

Also consider the following.

- Partner's current accounts are drawn up by the accountant (i.e. not a separate account, as if each partner had their own account within the business). They are likely to include, for example, postgraduate education allowance, seniority pay, etc. It is recommended that these accounts are zeroed each year. If a substantial amount builds up, the practice could go into the red if a partner was to leave and want that money.

- Getting professional help to go through the accounts with you (a specialist in GP finance and accountancy).

- Sources of private income (insurance certificates, medicals, sick notes, etc.).

- If a practice is doing well above or below average, why is this? Remember that if fraud is committed (i.e. too much is claimed), money will have to be reimbursed to the primary care trust. In this situation, all of the partners are liable.

Useful websites

Royal College of General Practitioners;
www.rcgp.org.uk

British Journal of General Practice;
www.rcgp.org.uk/rcgp/journal

British Medical Association;
www.bma.org.uk

British Medical Journal;
www.bmj.com

General Medical Council
www.gmc_uk.org

Bandolier (useful evidence-based reviews);
www.ebandolier.com

Cochrane Library;
www.cochranelibrary.com/cochrane

Prescribing database;
www.emims.net

Information educational resource, designed to support teaching and learning;
http://128.240.23.108/eprval/

Department of Health;
www.doh.gov.uk/dhhome.htm

GP-IK discussion group;
www.jiscmail.ac.uk/lists/gp-uk.html

JCPTGP;
www.jcptgp.org.uk

NHS Information Authority;
www.nhsia.nhs.uk

National electronic Library for Health;
www.nelh.nhs.uk

Search engine;
www.medisearch.co.uk

British National Formulary;
www.bnf.vhn.net

NHS Delivery Practice Database (interactive);
www.doh.gov.uk/learningzone/sdpinter.htm

NHS Beacon Programme run by The Modernisation Agency;
www.modernnhs.nhs.uk/nhsbeacons

HAZnet (Health Action Zones);
www.haznet.org.uk

National Institute for Mental Health in England;
www.doh.gov.uk/mentalhealth/nimhe.htm

Useful abbreviations

CHAI	Commission for Healthcare Audit and Inspection (took over from the Commission for Health Improvement in 2003)
CHI	Commission for Health Improvement
CHS	child health surveillance
CRHP	Council for the Regulation of Healthcare (oversees existing regulatory bodies)
DDA	Dispensing Doctors' Association
DHSS	Department of Health and Social Security
DSM	Diagnostic and Statistical Manual
FHSA	Family Health Services Authority
FPC	Family Practitioners' Committee (statutory body of the NHS)
GMC	General Medical Council
GMSC	General Medical Services Committee
GPC	General Practice Committee (previously GMSC)
GPFC	General Practice Finance Corporation
HA	Health authority

HImp   Health Improvement Programme
IOC   Interim Orders Committee (founded in 2000 to protect patients)
IOS   Items of service (part of General Medical Services)
LMC   Local Medical Committee
MAAG   Medical Audit Advisory Group
MHF   Mental Health Foundation
NANP   National Association of Non-Principals
NAO   National Audit Office
NCAA   National Clinical Assessment Authority
NHS   National Health Service
NICE   National Institute for Clinical Excellence
NPSA   National Patient Safety Agency
NSC   National Screening Committee
NSF   National Service Framework
ooh   Out of hours
PALS   Patient Advisory Liaison Service
PCG   Primary care group
PCT   Primary care trust
PGD   Patient Group Directive
PGEA   Postgraduate Education Allowance
PHLS   Public Health Laboratory Service
PIL   Patient information leaflet
PRIMIS   Primary Care Information Services
SEA   Significant event analysis
SIGN   Scottish Intercollegiate Guidelines Network
VTS   Vocational Training Scheme

Further reading

Books

- Warrell D, Cox TM, Firth JD and Benz EJ Jr (eds) (2003) *Oxford Textbook of Medicine* (4e). Oxford Medical Publications, Oxford.
- Souhami RL and Moxham J (eds) (2002) *Textbook of Medicine*. Churchill Livingstone, London.
- Johnson BE, Johnson CA, Murray JL and Apgar BS (1999) *Women's Health Care Handbook* (2e). Hanley and Belfus, Inc, Philadelphia, PA.
- Lissauer T and Clayden G (1996) *Illustrated Textbook of Paediatrics*. Mosby, London.
- Rughani A (2001) *The GP's Guide to Personal Development Plans* (2e). Radcliffe Medical Press, Oxford.
- Pendleton D and Hasler J (1997) *Professional Development in General Practice*. Oxford Medical Publications, Oxford.
- Lilley R, Davies G and Cain B (1999) *The PCG Team Builder: creating and maintaining effective team working. A workbook for the health service and primary care team*. Radcliffe Medical Press, Oxford.
- Arroba T and James K (1992) *Pressure at Work: a practical survival guide for all managers* (2e). McGraw-Hill Education, Maidenhead.

- Palmer KT (1997) *Notes for the MRCGP* (3e). Blackwell Science, Oxford.
- Petrie A (1987) *Lecture Notes on Medical Statistics* (2e). Blackwell Scientific Publications, Oxford.
- Fentem R (2000) *Discovering Advanced Mathematics*. Collins Educational, London.
- Greenhalgh T (2000) *How to Read a Paper: the basics of evidence-based medicine*. BMJ Publishing Group, London.
- Clark R and Croft P (1998) *Critical Reading for the Reflective Practitioner: a guide to primary care*. Butterworth Heinemann, Oxford.
- Stacey E and Toun Y (1997) *Critical Reading Questions for the MRCGP*. BIOS Scientific Publishers, Oxford.
- Gardiner P, Chana N and Jones R (2001) *An Insider's Guide to the MRCGP Oral Exam*. Radcliffe Medical Press, Oxford.

Journals and periodicals

- *Pulse*
- *Update*
- *GP*
- *Doctor*
- *Practitioner*
- *Medeconomics*

Index